Practical Procedures in the Management of Tooth Wear

Practical Procedures in the Management of Tooth Wear

Subir Banerji BDS, MClinDent(Prostho), PhD, MFGDP(UK), FDS RCPS(Glasg), FICOI, FICD FIADFE
Dental Practitioner, Programme Director MSc Aesthetic Dentistry
Senior Clinical Lecturer, King's College London, Faculty of Dentistry, Oral & Craniofacial Sciences, Private Practice, London, UK

Shamir Mehta BDS, BSc, MClinDent(Prosth), FFGDP(UK), FDS RCPS (Glasg), FDS RCS (Eng), FICD
Dental Practitioner, Senior Clinical Lecturer, King's College London, Faculty of Oral & Craniofacial Sciences/Deputy Programme Director MSc Aesthetic Dentistry, Private Practice Middlesex, London, UK;
Undertaking research at Radboud University Medical Center, Radboud Institute for Health Sciences, Department of Dentistry, Nijmegen, The Netherlands

Niek Opdam DDS, PhD
Associate Professor, Radboud University Medical Center, Radboud Institute for Health Sciences, Department of Dentistry, Nijmegen;
Dental Practitioner in Adhesive Dentistry, Tandzorg Ulft, The Netherlands

Bas Loomans DDS, PhD
Assistant Professor, Radboud University Medical Center, Radboud Institute for Health Sciences, Department of Dentistry, Nijmegen;
Dental Practitioner, Mondzorg Oost, Nijmegen, The Netherlands

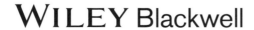
WILEY Blackwell

This edition first published 2020
© 2020 John Wiley & Sons Ltd

The right of Subir Banerji, Shamir Mehta, Niek Opdam and Bas Loomans to be identified as the authors of this work has been asserted in accordance with law.

Registered Offices   John Wiley & Sons, Inc., 111 River Street, Hoboken, NJ 07030, USA
John Wiley & Sons Ltd, The Atrium, Southern Gate, Chichester, West Sussex, PO19 8SQ, UK

Editorial Office   9600 Garsington Road, Oxford, OX4 2DQ, UK

For details of our global editorial offices, customer services, and more information about Wiley products visit us at www.wiley.com.

Wiley also publishes its books in a variety of electronic formats and by print-on-demand. Some content that appears in standard print versions of this book may not be available in other formats.

Library of Congress Cataloging-in-Publication Data

Names: Banerji, Subir, 1961– author. | Mehta, Shamir B., author. |
    Opdam, Niek, 1956– author. | Loomans, Bas, 1974– author.
Title: Practical procedures in the management of tooth wear / Subir Banerji,
    Shamir Mehta, Niek Opdam, Bas Loomans.
Description: Hoboken, NJ : Wiley-Blackwell, 2020. |
    Includes bibliographical references and index.
Identifiers: LCCN 2019026465 (print) | ISBN 9781119389866 (paperback) |
    ISBN 9781119389842 (adobe pdf) | ISBN 9781119389927 (epub)
Subjects: MESH: Tooth Wear–therapy | Tooth Wear–diagnosis
Classification: LCC RK340 (print) | LCC RK340 (ebook) | NLM WU 166 | DDC 617.6/34–dc23
LC record available at https://lccn.loc.gov/2019026465
LC ebook record available at https://lccn.loc.gov/2019026466

Cover Design: Wiley
Cover Images: Subir Banerji, Shamir Mehta, Niek Opdam and Bas Loomans

Set in 10/12pt Warnock by SPi Global, Pondicherry, India
Printed and bound in Singapore by Markono Print Media Pte Ltd

10 9 8 7 6 5 4 3 2 1

Contents

Foreword

Tooth wear (TW) is increasing throughout the world, potentially because of factors such as increased consumption of carbonated drinks, bruxism, and the increasing prevalence of gastric regurgitation. In the past, the treatment of TW has been considered to be the domain of the specialist restorative dentist, and, in the distant past, treatment involved crowning teeth afflicted by wear, surely a grossly inappropriate way to treat already compromised teeth. However, contemporary techniques using resin composite, alongside improvements in dentine bonding agents, have brought about the genesis of a new, minimally invasive treatment regimen. Such a technique generally involves coverage of worn and wearing surfaces by resin composite placed at an increased occlusal vertical dimension, provided that the patient understands the short-term disadvantages, such as being unable to chew on the discluded posterior teeth, potential for lisping because of the change in shape of the restored anterior teeth, and the occasional loss or chipping of the restorations.

This book presents a comprehensive examination of all aspects of the causes and extent of TW, alongside minimally invasive methods for treatment, written by a group of clinicians who have extensive experience in the field. It says it as it is – 'management of a patient presenting with TW is by no means always a straightforward matter', adding that 'as patients are increasingly presenting with signs of tooth wear to their general dental practitioner, the latter should acquire the necessary skills and knowledge to treat this in the primary care setting'. This book therefore sets the scene by comprehensively discussing the cases of TW, before moving on to describe clinical assessment and diagnosis (including noteworthy medical conditions, principally, gastric disorders) and a comprehensive section on the patient examination and an equally comprehensive section on the aesthetic zone and the indices which might be helpful in recording the patient's condition. Chapter 5 covers occlusion in depth before moving on to the Dahl concept and describes the relative axial tooth movement that is observed when a localised appliance or localised restorations are placed in supra-occlusion and the occlusion re-establishes full-arch contacts over a period of time. This concept is central to contemporary techniques for treatment of TW, being the concept of 'additive' rather than 'subtractive' treatment, with the former being easier for the patient and clinician alike.

This appropriately titled book *Practical Procedures in the Management of Tooth Wear* devotes five chapters to an in-depth review of treatment methodology, clearly describing the materials and techniques which are employed and why they are employed, alongside a wealth of appropriate illustrations. It also includes many technique tips for clinicians who wish to become involved in treatment of TW, not only on anterior teeth but also posterior teeth, also presenting the variety of means at clinicians' disposal. Of course, there is no point in describing 'how to do it' in the absence of information on the potential for success of treatment. Chapter 14 describes this, leaving the reader in no doubt that the minimally invasive theme throughout the book is on the right track.

The authors are to be congratulated on the clarity of their writing and their illustrations, and the array of references provides the evidence to back up their statements. The icing on the cake for readers is their access to nine valuable videos supplementing, 'live', many of the clinical techniques and aspects of TW described in the text. This comprehensive text on all aspects of the pathogenesis, diagnosis, and treatment of TW is therefore very much to be welcomed, given that it can facilitate the way for primary care dentists, indeed for all dentists, to demystify the treatment of this increasingly common condition.

Professor F.J. Trevor Burke, *BDS, MDS, DDS, MSc, MGDS, FDS RCS,*
(Edin.), FDS RCS (Eng.), FFGDP(UK), FADM
Professor of Primary Dental Care
Honorary Consultant in Restorative Dentistry in the
Institute of Clinical Sciences
The School of Dentistry
Birmingham University
Birmingham, UK

Acknowledgement

An endeavour such as this is never an individual effort. This book was conceptually realised about six years ago and has been taking shape ever since. We wanted to articulate in an easy-to-understand manner the complex and sometimes controversial contemporary management of tooth wear, which is recognised as a universal clinical problem by colleagues all over the world.

Credit must be given to our own teachers, past and present, along with our research collaborations and students, amongst whom many discussions have taken place to develop the material for this publication.

Our families have supported us tirelessly and with the utmost patience, through the many hours which were spent assimilating the text and videos. We are indebted to our patients who have so kindly agreed to show stages of their treatment to enable us to illustrate the techniques and protocols which we have advocated in this book. Thank you to Dr Krisanth Ragudhas for the editing and production of many of the videos that accompany the text. Staff at our publisher, Wiley, have been patient and supportive. We sincerely hope that our efforts will benefit our colleagues and students when they are treating and managing their patients with the signs and symptoms of tooth wear.

Subir, Shamir, Niek, and Bas

About the Companion Website

Don't forget to visit the companion website for this book:

www.wiley.com/go/banerji/toothwear

There you will find valuable material designed to enhance your learning, including:

- Hours of high-quality videos demonstrating clinical techniques and procedures.

Scan this QR code to visit the companion website.

1

Introduction and the Prevalence of Tooth Wear

1.1 Introduction

There are increasing concerns over the levels of non-carious tooth surface loss being encountered amongst patients attending for routine dental examinations in general dental practice.[1] Indeed due to its prevalence, it has become common practice (in at least some countries) to carry out risk assessments for the presence of tooth wear (TW) as part of the overall process of performing the accepted assessments and evaluations during a dental examination.[2]

Given the frequent and varied range of physical, mechanical, and chemical challenges faced by human dentition on a daily basis, the irreversible wearing-away of the dental hard tissues can be assumed to most likely occur as a result of the natural ageing process. Consequently, TW is a 'normal' physiological process and differs somewhat from a number of the other oral diseases that are also routinely screened for such as dental caries, periodontal disease or oral mucosal conditions, which are all by definition pathological processes. Difficulty may, however, be encountered in attempting to determine the clinical distinction between TW that may be considered representative of the consequences of the natural ageing process, commonly referred to as physiological wear, and an appearance worthy of a diagnostic entity. It is therefore important to consider some of the key terms and definitions in relation to the irreversible wearing-away of tooth tissue, and to further explore some of the ambiguities and confusion that surrounds the application of these terms.

The term *tooth wear (TW)* is a general term that can be used to describe the surface loss of dental hard tissues from causes other than dental caries or dental trauma.[3] Usually, TW is subdivided into subforms, such as *attrition, abrasion,* and *erosion,* in accordance with the suspected/known aetiology. Whilst these aetiological factors can sometimes occur in isolation, clinically it is difficult (if not at times impossible) to identify a single causative factor when a patient presents with TW as the condition more often than not has a multifactorial aetiology. For this reason, the term *tooth surface loss (TSL)* was suggested by Eccles in 1982 to embrace all of the aetiological factors regardless of whether the exact cause of wear has been identified.[4]

Given the above, the authors have a preference towards a subdivision that indicates that there is a combination of factors that lead to tissue loss. Accordingly,

Practical Procedures in the Management of Tooth Wear, First Edition. Subir Banerji, Shamir Mehta, Niek Opdam and Bas Loomans.
© 2020 John Wiley & Sons Ltd. Published 2020 by John Wiley & Sons Ltd.
Companion website: www.wiley.com/go/banerji/toothwear

the nature of dental wear may be broadly divided into *mechanical wear* and *chemical wear,* and both forms further subdivided into *intrinsic and extrinsic,* with the overall existence of four subforms, hence:

- *mechanical intrinsic TW* (as a result of chewing or bruxism, also called *attrition*)
- *mechanical extrinsic TW* (due to factors other than chewing and/or bruxism, also called *abrasion*, for example with a toothbrush)
- *chemical intrinsic TW* (as consequence of gastric acid, also called *erosion*)
- *chemical extrinsic dental wear* (as a result of an acidic diet, also known as *erosion*).

Unfortunately, there is considerable ambiguity with the application of some of the above terms (nationally and internationally) that renders effective communication between healthcare providers challenging, especially when attempting to draw comparisons between differing items of dental research.

It had been proposed by Smith et al.[5] that the use of the term TSL may inadvertently imply an under-estimation of the actual extent and severity of the problem by suggesting the condition to only refer to the surface (or superficial) loss of tooth tissue (as opposed to the additional subsurface loss), which is often seen clinically, thereby failing to take into account cases of more extensive tooth tissue loss. Consequently, they have suggested that the use of the term TW be preferred where there may be inadequate evidence to strongly support the cause of wear being a result of erosion, attrition or abrasion (so as to facilitate the process of communication between dentists and with their patients).[5] As a result, the authors do not recommend use of the term *erosive tooth wear* (as is often evidenced in many scientific publications), as this implies that erosion is the primary aetiological factor.

1.2   Physiological Wear and Pathological Wear: The Concept of Severe Tooth Wear

It has been suggested that as teeth continue to function and thus remain continually exposed to erosive, abrasive, and attritive factors, the wearing-away of tooth tissue will probably occur as an age-related phenomenon.[6]

A number of reports have been published describing the rates of TW progression. Lambrechts et al. have estimated the normal vertical loss of enamel from physiological wear to be approximately 18 μm for premolar teeth and 38 μm for molar teeth, respectively, per annum.[7] Comparable rates of progression have been reported in a more recent study by Rodriguez et al.[8] With specific reference to incisor teeth, by the means of undertaking a cross-sectional digital radiographic study to estimate the rate of incisor TW amongst 346 subjects Ray et al. have reported the average crown height of a maxillary central incisor to decrease by 1.01 mm (approximately 1000 μm) from 11.94 mm between the age of 10 years to 70 years, and for mandibular central incisor teeth, the average crown height to decrease by 1.46 mm (approximately 1500 μm) to 9.58 mm over a period of six decades (when applying the same age ranges), representing the mean annual wear rates of central incisor teeth to be in the range of 17–25 µm per year of life.[9]

The term *physiological wear* (Figure 1.1) is thus commonly applied to describe that level of TW observed which is expected for the patient's age, commensurate with normal day-to-day function.[10]

Historically the term *pathological wear* (Figure 1.2a–d) was used to relate to the presence of unacceptable wear for a particular age group based on clinical judgement and has been traditionally applied as describing a level of wear when restorative intervention may be justified. However, the use of clinical judgement clearly does not permit an accurate and consistent approach as this would require the concomitant need to define the precise 'normal levels of wear' (that should be present in differing age groups and populations), as well as the availability of a reasonably accurate and consistent method to measure the levels of wear actually present. Given the current lack of knowledge in relation to the pathogenesis of TW (with two common theories being described, one of slow cumulative progression occurring throughout life – often referred to as *continual* and the alternative of cyclical bursts of activity – commonly termed *episodic*),[6] it would be very difficult to determine meaningful benchmark values for the levels of TW likely to be present amongst individuals of differing ages.[6]

In 2017, in an attempt to improve clarity and understating, the term *pathological wear* was defined in a European Consensus Statement on the Management Guidelines (for Severe Wear) as 'tooth wear which is atypical for the age of the patient causing pain or discomfort, functional problems, or deterioration of aesthetic appearance, which if it progresses, may give rise to undesirable complications of increased complexity'.[11] However, ambiguity is still likely to remain for the reasons discussed above.

It has therefore been suggested that the diagnostic entity of *severe tooth wear* may be more appropriate when undertaking clinical assessments. The latter term has been defined as 'tooth wear with substantial loss of tooth structure, with dentine exposure and significant loss (more than or equal to one third) of the clinical crown'.[11] The presence of severe wear can be used to define the highest grade of a clinical index, which in turn may be used to screen for the extent and severity of TW present, in a manner similar to other indices and monitoring tools used in clinical dentistry (Figure 1.3).

However, the use of an index based on the severity of TW observed clinically may be of limited merit in identifying treatment need. This can be illustrated by the example of the case of a young patient, seen in Figure 1.4, diagnosed with erosive pathological TW on the palatal surfaces of the maxillary central incisor teeth by virtue of the level of wear clinically present. In addition there are symptoms of sensitivity and an aesthetic impairment. However, with the absence of less than one-third clinical crown loss, severe wear (by definition) may not be present in this case, although active restorative intervention would likely be indicated. In contrast, signs of severe wear may be seen to exist in an 89-year-old (see Figure 1.5), but in this case there would be no clear indication to provide any forms of active restorative intervention.

The use of indices for TW is discussed further in Chapter 3.

1.3 The Prevalence of TW

In relation to the matter of the prevalence of TW (amongst adult dentate patients), the 2009 UK Adult Dental Health Survey (ADHS) reported:[12]

- 77% of the 6469 adults examined showed some signs of TW in the anterior teeth (compared with 66% in 1989), with the type of wear described as being consistent with normal ageing with the exposure of dentine on the incisal tips
- 15% displayed signs of moderate wear (presenting with more extensive dentine exposure) and 2% severe TW (with the level of presenting hard tissue wear extending as far as secondary dentine)
- the damage was cumulative, with an increased prevalence with age and with more than 80% of the over-50-year-olds exhibiting some TW, but an increasing proportion of moderate wear amongst younger adults – likely to be clinically important
- TW was more prevalent amongst males (71% versus 61% for females)
- signs of moderate TW increased by 4% between 1998 (11%) and 2009 (15%)
- although severe TW remains relatively rare, the incidence had increased since the previous survey in 1998.

Given an ageing Western population retaining its natural teeth into advanced years, supported by a progressive decline in the number of edentulous patients as highlighted in the 2009 UK ADHS (with a 22% reduction in the proportion of such patients since 1978), it is hardly surprising to see signs of TW amongst older patients. Such teeth will have been exposed to a plethora of elements that may lead to wear by intrinsic and extrinsic factors over a sustained period spanning several decades.

As part of a systematic review of the results of 186 prevalence studies of TW by all causes, it was concluded that the percentage of adult patients presenting with severe TW increased from 3% at the age of 20 years to 17% at the age of 70 years, with a tendency to develop more wear with age.[13] The results of a large epidemiological study amongst German dental patients reported similar results, where the extent of TW was scored on a scale from 0 to 3 (with higher scores indicating more severe levels of TW), with mean wear scores increasing from 0.6 amongst 20–29 year olds to 1.4 in 70–79 year olds.[14]

There also seem to be variations in the incidence rates of TW amongst patients residing in different European countries, with the highest level of wear rates being reported in the UK.[15] The latter has been possibly accounted for by risk factors such as heartburn, acid reflux, repeated vomiting, and acidic intake, especially related to the consumption of fresh fruit and isotonic/energy drinks (as discussed further in Chapter 3). This study also showed approximately 30% of the subjects to demonstrate visible signs of TW, with evidence of a moderate rise in TW with increasing age, and a prevalence of severe wear being reported amongst 3% of the subjects included.

Whilst the criteria applied for identifying and scoring TW show wide variation amongst different studies, there has been considerable interest in studies documenting the prevalence of erosive TW, as it would appear that there has been a considerable increase in the incidence of erosion-related TW amongst children and young adults over the course of the past three decades.

Erosion was initially included in the UK Children's Dental Health Survey in 1993.[16] When reassessed in 1996/1997, a trend towards a higher prevalence of erosion in children aged between 3.5 years and 4.5 years (Figure 1.6) was identified (particularly amongst those children who consumed carbonated drinks on an almost daily basis when compared to toddlers consuming these drinks less frequently).[17] The initial Child Dental Health Survey also reported 25% of 11-year-olds and 32% of 14-year-olds assessed in their sample as showing signs of erosion affecting the palatal surfaces of their maxillary incisor teeth (which in more severe cases had progressed to involve the dentinal tissues and in some cases the pulp complex). It also revealed that almost half of the 5- and 6-year-olds studied demonstrated signs of erosion affecting the primary dentition, with almost 25% showing signs of dentinal or pulpal tissue involvement.

In another extensive UK-based study in 2004, in which 1753 children were examined at the age of 12 years and observed for a period of two years thereafter, 59.7% were reported to have evidence of TW at the commencement of the study, of which 2.7% had dentine exposure, which rose to 8.9% over the course of the two-year observation period.[18]

In the Netherlands, a survey amongst 622 children performed by El Aidi et al.[19] found that significant erosive wear was present in 1.8% of the 11-year-olds and 23.8% of the 15-year-olds. The incidence of new tooth surfaces exhibiting erosive wear, in erosion-free children, decreased significantly with age. In children with tooth erosion the condition progressed steadily. Therefore, it is likely that TW is an increasing problem amongst younger individuals but limited to specific risk groups.[20]

Erosive TW is caused by acidic substrates that may be either of an intrinsic origin or an extrinsic source. The consumption of soft drinks in the UK has been reported to have increased by sevenfold between the 1950s and 1990s, with adolescents and children accounting for 65% of all purchases, and a per capita intake of 15 l per person.[21] Likewise, soft drink consumption has also been reported to have increased in the USA by 300% over a period of 20 years, with serving sizes increasing from 185 g in the 1950s to 570 g in the late 1990s.[22] Table 1.1 lists the typical pH values of some commonly consumed beverages, as well as details of some of the acidic content.

Table 1.1 The pH values of commonly consumed beverages.

Beverage	Type	pH value (SD)
Pepsi-Cola	Diet	3.02 (0.01)
Coca Cola	Classic	2.37 (0.03)
Coca Cola	Caffeine-free, diet	3.04 (0.01
Red Bull	Sugar Free	3.39 (0.00)
Fanta	Orange	2.82 (0.02)
Orange juice	Minute Maid	3.82 (0.01)
Orangeade	Minute Maid	2.85 (0.00)

Other factors which may be responsible for the high rates of erosive TW described by the above studies include regurgitation, which may be either involuntary, associated with conditions such as hiatus hernia, or voluntary, as seen amongst patients presenting with eating disorders such as anorexia nervosa or bulimia nervosa.[23] Dental erosion may also be induced by environmental influences, such as that seen amongst those workers exposed to acids in the workplace.

A knowledge of the at-risk groups can help to target treatment and, in particular, preventative care. However, targeting at-risk groups is challenging in itself, as no clear definitions have been described. Given the effects of erosive damage on the permanent dentition of teenagers and younger adults, with the increased risk for needing repetitive and invariably costly restorative care, the importance of focussing on and delivering effective prevention for such groups is further highlighted, and is discussed in more detail in Chapter 7.

1.4 An Overview of the Challenges Associated with TW

The management of a patient presenting with TW is by no means always a straightforward matter, often requiring specialist attention where complex restorative care may be indicated for more severe cases. However, given that patients are increasingly presenting with signs of tooth tissue loss to their general dental practitioner, it is likely that the latter will have to acquire the necessary skills and knowledge to effectively care for and provide appropriate management in the primary care setting.

Aspects that may compound difficulties associated with TW management include:[24]

- the general lack of widespread awareness of TW amongst the public
- the lack of knowledge concerning the pathogenesis of TW
- challenges associated with deriving an accurate diagnosis, inclusive of the limitation of the available diagnostic methods and the confusion surrounding key diagnostic terms
- how to best deliver effective preventative care and implement monitoring strategies
- uncertainties in knowing at which precise stage to implement active restorative intervention (as opposed to simple passive management and monitoring strategy)
- a lack of understanding on how to predictably restore such severely worn dentitions, with the aim of ultimately attaining a functionally and aesthetically stable restored dentition
- a lack of knowledge relating to the availability of contemporary materials and their respective techniques of application.

These matters will be addressed in this textbook and the accompanying videos.

1.5 Conclusion

A clear understanding of the terminology, prevalence, and aetiological factors associated with TW is an important prerequisite to developing an effective strategy to manage patients who present with this condition. Subsequent chapters and the videos will elaborate further on the various aspects relevant to this topic.

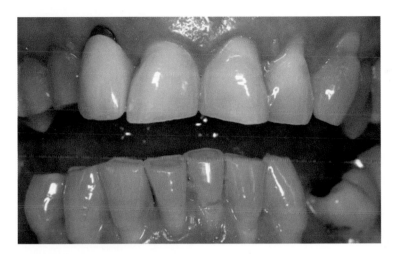

Figure 1.1 Physiological TW in a 76-year-old male.

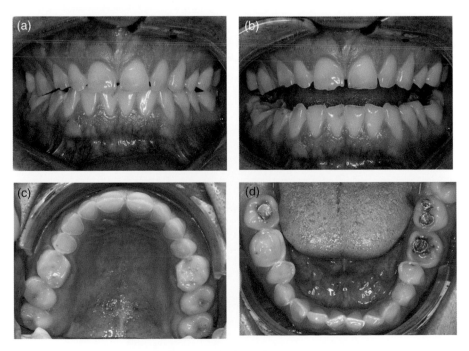

Figure 1.2 A patient in his mid-30s with pathological TW.

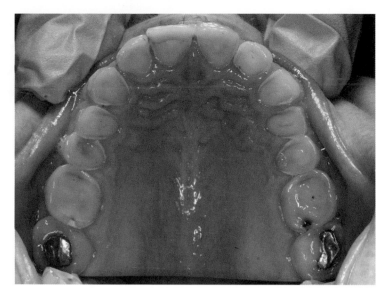

Figure 1.3 The upper teeth shown in a patient with severe TW. There is substantial loss of tooth structure, with dentine exposure and significant loss (more than or equal to one-third) of the clinical crown seen in the premolars and the upper first molars.

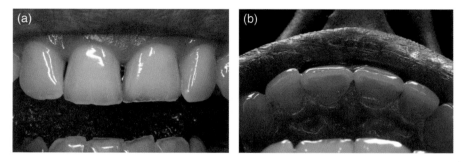

Figure 1.4 Pathological TW affecting the palatal surfaces of the upper central incisors. Patient complains of an aesthetic impairment and tooth sensitivity from these central incisors.

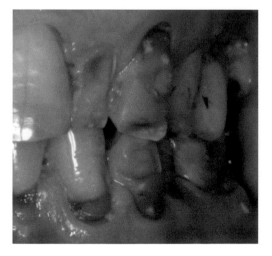

Figure 1.5 Severe TW depicted in this 89-year-old patient on the upper left lateral incisor and canine teeth.

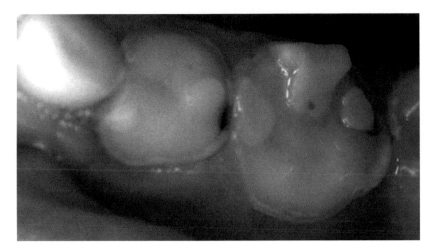

Figure 1.6 Erosive TW in the primary dentition.

References

1 Meyers, I.A. (2013). Minimum intervention dentistry and the management of tooth wear in general dental practice. *Aust. Dent. Jour.* 58 (1 (Suppl)): 60–65.
2 (2016). *Clinical Examination & Record Keeping, Good Practice Guidelines*, 3e. FGDP(UK): Hadden AM.
3 Yule, P. and Barclay, S. (2015). Worn dentition by toothwear? Aetiology, diagnosis and management revisited. *Dent. Update* 42: 525–532.
4 Eccles, J. (1982). Tooth surface loss from abrasion, attrition and erosion. *Dent. Update* 9: 373–381.
5 (a) Smith, B.G., Bartlett, D.W., and Robb, N.D. (1997). The prevalence, etiology and management of tooth wear in the United Kingdom. *J. Prosthet. Dent.* 78 (4): 367–372.
  (b) Hattab, F. and Yassin, O. Etiology and diagnosis of tooth wear: a literature review and presentation of selected cases. *Int. J. Prosthodont.* 20 (13): 101–107.
6 Bartlett, W. and Dugmore, C. (2008). Pathological or physiological erosion – is there a relationship to age? *Clin. Oral Investig.* (Suppl 1): S27–S31.
7 Lamberechts, P., Braeme, M., Vuylsteke-Wauters, M., and Vanherle, G. (1989). Quantitative in vivo wear of human enamel. *J. Dent. Res.* 68: 1752–1754.
8 Rodgriguez, J., Austin, R., and Bartlett, D. (2012). In vivo measurements of tooth wear over 12 months. *Caries Res.* 46: 9–15.
9 Ray, D., Weiman, A., Patel, P. et al. (2015). Estimation of the rate of tooth wear in permanent incisors: a cross sectional digital radiographic study. *J. Oral Rehabil.* 42: 460–466.
10 Burke, F. and McKenna, G. (2011). Toothwear and the older patient. *Dent. Update* 38 (3): 165–168.
11 Loomans, B., Opdam, N., Attin, T. et al. (2017). Severe tooth wear: European consensus statement on management guidelines. *J. Adhes. Dent.* 19: 111–119.
12 (2011). *UK Adult Dental Health Survey 2009*. The Health and Social Care Information Centre.

13 Van't Spijker, A., Kreulen, C., and Bartlett, D. (2009). Prevalence of tooth wear in adults. *Int. J. Prosthodont.* 22: 35–42.

14 Bernhardt, O., Gesch, D., Splieth, D. et al. (2004). Risk factors for high occlusal wear scores in a population based sample: results of the study of health in Pomerania (SHIP). *Int. J. Prosthodont.* 17: 333–337.

15 Bartlett, D., Lussi, A., West, N. et al. (2013). Prevalence of tooth wear on buccal and lingual surfaces and possible risk factors in young European adults. *J. Dent.* 41: 1007–1013.

16 O'Brien, M. (1993). *Childrens dental health in the UK*, 74–76. HMSO. 1994.

17 Lussi, A., Hellwig, G., Zero, D., and Jaeggi, T. (2006). Erosive tooth wear: diagnosis, risk factors and prevalence. *Am. J. Dent.* 19: 319–325.

18 Dugmore, C. and Rock, W. (2003). Awareness of tooth erosion in 12 year old children by primary dental care practitioners. *Community Dent. Health* 20: 223–227.

19 El Aidi, H., Bronkhorst, E.M., Huysmans, M.C., and Truin, G.J. (2010 Feb). Dynamics of tooth erosion in adolescents: a 3-year longitudinal study. *J. Dent.* 38 (2): 131–137.

20 Wetselaar, P., Vermaire, J.H., Visscher, C.M. et al. (2016). The prevalence of tooth wear in the Dutch adult population. *Caries Res.* 50: 543–550.

21 Shaw, L. and Smith, A. (1994). Erosion in children. An increasing clinical problem? *Dent. Update* 21: 103–106.

22 Calvadini, C., Siega-Riz, A., and Popkin, B. (2000). US adolescent food intake trends form 1965 to 1996. *Arch. Dis. Child.* 83: 18–24.

23 Kelleher, M. and Bishop, K. (2000). Tooth surface loss: an overview. Article 1. In: *Tooth Surface Loss*, 3–7. BDJ Books.

24 Mehta, S.B., Banerji, S., Millar, B.J., and Saurez-Feito, J.M. (2012). Current concepts on the management of tooth wear: Part 1. Assessment, treatment planning and strategies for the prevention and passive management of tooth wear. *Br. Dent. J.* 212: 17–27.

2

The Aetiology and Presentation of Tooth Wear

2.1   Introduction

It is generally accepted that tooth wear (TW) has a multifactorial nature. Whilst there are a variety of established cofactors that may exacerbate the process of TW (such as hyposalivation and hypomineralisation),[1] there are a number of primary mechanisms (which although themselves are neither descriptive of the wear process nor infer direct causation)[2] that serve to provide an account of the clinical outcomes of a variety of occurrences where the experience of and/or exposure to specific factors or elements may produce the observed clinical patterns of TW.

As discussed in Chapter 1, the nature of dental wear may be divided into *mechanical wear* and *chemical wear*. Both forms can be further subdivided into *intrinsic* and *extrinsic*. There are therefore four subforms: *mechanical intrinsic tooth wear* (as a result of chewing or bruxism, also called attrition), *mechanical extrinsic tooth wear* (due to factors other than chewing and/or bruxism, also called abrasion), *chemical intrinsic tooth wear* (as consequence of gastric acid, also called erosion), and *chemical extrinsic dental wear* (as a result of an acidic diet, also known as erosion).

When attempting to manage a worn dentition, the identification of the various aetiological factors associated with TW for that particular patient is a critical stage to the overall success of the treatment plan. Knowledge of the aetiological factors will allow for the preparation of an appropriate preventative protocol. The aim for this would be to halt, or significantly curtail, the actions and consequences of the various aetiological factors for which the patient must not only assume responsibility, but also fully understand the consequences of failing to do so.[1]

However, given the multifactorial origin of TW, the establishment of an accurate diagnosis of the aetiological factors can sometimes prove highly challenging.[3] The mechanisms cited above may result in the development of clinically distinguishable characteristics, given the nature of TW (often involving several factors and sometimes cofactors acting with differing levels of intensity and effect), however the appearance of such lesions may not always provide firm clues as to *all* of the likely aetiological factors involved but may give an indication of the predominant aetiological factor responsible. This places an emphasis on the need to take a meticulous oral history, often involving the use of questionnaires

Practical Procedures in the Management of Tooth Wear, First Edition. Subir Banerji, Shamir Mehta, Niek Opdam and Bas Loomans.
© 2020 John Wiley & Sons Ltd. Published 2020 by John Wiley & Sons Ltd.
Companion website: www.wiley.com/go/banerji/toothwear

such as the Oral Health Impact Profile (OHIP),[4] which can be used to evaluate the oral health-related quality of life of patients with severe TW, as discussed further in Chapter 3.

The OHIP is the most frequently used oral-specific measure for oral health-related quality of life. It is a questionnaire that contains 49 statements organised in seven domains: functional limitation, physical pain, psychological discomfort, physical disability, psychological disability, social disability, and handicap. The validity and reliability of the original English version of the OHIP have been evaluated in several epidemiological and cross-cultural studies.[5,6]

For specific problems regarding appearance, a separate questionnaire has also been developed, the Orofacial Esthetic Scale (OES), which aims to obtain a characterisation of the orofacial aesthetics.[7,8]

2.2 Intrinsic Mechanical Wear

Intrinsic mechanical wear, also called *attrition* may be considered as *the wearing-away of tooth structure as a result of tooth-to-tooth contact*. It is thus usually observed to involve the occlusal and incisal contacting surfaces, and perhaps less frequently observed to occur on the axial surfaces (where, for instance, an anomalous type of malocclusion may be seen to exist).[9]

Whilst wear by attrition will occur as part of the natural ageing process, the rate of wear as a result of tooth-to-tooth contact may be accelerated by several further mechanical and chemical factors, including:[9]

- parafunctional tooth clenching and grinding habits (bruxism)
- a coarse or acidic diet
- intrinsic acids (reflux)
- abrasive dust
- a traumatic occlusion in the case of a patient with several missing teeth
- the presence of an anterior open bite, crossbite or an edge-to-edge incisor relationship.

It is not uncommon for patients to present in general practice with signs suggestive of a tendency towards parafunctional habits often complaining of temporomandibular disorder (TMD),[1,10] where anecdotal connections are routinely made between the presence of such tendencies and that of a wearing dentition. However, it would appear that there exists only limited evidence in the contemporary literature to actually support the role of bruxing activity alone (in the absence of erosive factors) as a major cause of TW.[2] Indeed, the results of a study by Smith and Knight in 1984 reported that the mechanism of erosion had a likely role in the aetiology of TW seen amongst 89% of the patients.[11]

In relation to the appearance of lesions likely to be formed as a result of the mechanism of attrition during the formative stage, the clinical manifestation may typically comprise a small polished facet on the cusp or ridge, or the slight flattening of an incisal edge. With progression, however, lesions due to attritional wear often demonstrate the tendency towards the reduction of the cusp height and flattening of the occlusal inclined planes, with concomitant dentine exposure.[2,9]

The presence of dentine exposure (given its physico-chemical differences with enamel tissue) is likely to result in an increase in the rate of wear. With increased levels of dentine exposure, it would not be uncommon for patients to attend complaining of tooth sensitivity to a variety of stimuli. However, where the rate of TW may be relatively slow and evenly progressive, dentine hypersensitivity is seldom reported due to the formation of secondary dentine. In the later stages, teeth affected by the process of attritional wear may display a marked shortening of the clinical crown height.[9,12]

Figure 2.1 illustrates severe wear where the pattern of wear has a likely attritional component (based on the taking of an accurate patient history).

2.3 Extrinsic Mechanical Wear

Extrinsic mechanical wear is caused by contact with extrinsic factors not involving tooth-to-tooth contact. This wear is often called *abrasion*, and the most common causes are oral habits such as brushing habits, biting nails, pens, and pencils, and coming into contact with the mouthpieces of music instruments, as well as intraoral piercings.

It is generally accepted that the most common cause of dental abrasion in the cervical portion of a tooth/teeth is likely to be due to improper toothbrushing technique (often related to the activity of overzealous or vigorous practice, the time and frequency of brushing, bristle design) and/or the use of abrasive dentifrices. There are also some clinical manifestations of abrasive wear that may relate to a given habit (where the taking of a clear and accurate patient history may prove pivotal in establishing the likely cause). These include:[13]

- the asymmetric notching of incisal edges that can result from a habit of pipe smoking, nut/seed cracking (such as watermelon and pumpkin seeds) or nail biting (Figure 2.2)
- the notching of teeth from occupational associated habits, for example amongst carpenters, hairdressers and tailors where they may be utilising their teeth to hold nails, hairclips and tacks, respectively, where the pattern will likely be irregular and will usually relate to the area of the mouth used and the frequency of the habit
- wear amongst musicians using their teeth to grip onto the mouthpieces of various instruments
- the chewing of abrasive materials such as sand, or environmental exposure to dust in the workplace such as amongst iron-works, mines, and quarries
- proximal root abrasion due to the inappropriate use of dental floss or toothpicks, or iatrogenic activity including the improper use of a dental bur or abrasive strip or polishing medium
- wear from antagonistic porcelain-based restorations[10]
- labial wear that may sometimes be caused by brushing with sodium bicarbonate powder.[9]

Abrasive lesions related to toothbrushing can sometimes be unilateral (whereby left-sided lesions are more likely to be seen amongst right-handed patients)[14] and are typified by the presence of rounded or V-shaped notches seen on the buccal/labial surfaces in the region of the cement–enamel junction (where the dentine and cementum tissues offer a lower resistance to wear than enamel).[9] Canine and premolar teeth seem to be most commonly affected.[9] The role of acid exposure at or about the time of toothbrushing (within 1 hour) may also have a role in the initiation and progression of TW lesions by abrasion.[13]

Figure 2.3 shows an example of the classical pattern of abrasive wear due to overzealous toothbrushing activity.

2.4 Non-carious Cervical Lesions

Whilst TW on the occlusal, buccal, and palatal surfaces due to mechanical and chemical wear etiological factors is widely accepted as a process exhibiting in patients over time, specific wear located at the cervical enamel–cement junction is more difficult to explain. These cervical lesions have been traditionally explained as caused by too vigorous brushing habits but in the 1990s the explanative diagnosis of *abfraction* emerged, indicating that occlusal forces and consequently bending of teeth played a role in cervical tooth substance loss.

Abfraction is defined as 'the loss of hard tissue from eccentric occlusal loads leading to compressive and tensile stresses at the cervical fulcrum area of the tooth. The tensile stresses weaken the cervical hydroxyapetitie, which produces a special form of wedge shaped defect with sharp rims at the cemeto-enamel junction.'[15] The repetitive displacement of cervical restorations has been suggested to occur as a result of this concept (also sometimes termed *stress-induced cervical lesions* or *cervical stress lesions*).[14]

As discussed above, there is a lack of consensus surrounding the actual existence of this concept, which has been described in the literature as perhaps being of a merely hypothetical nature (due to the lack of substantial evidence to support the existence of this concept), with toothbrush-dentifrice abrasion or acid erosion being cited as the likely cause of such forms of TW.[16] It has been argued that aggressive toothbrushing techniques cannot account for some of the observations that can be described or indeed have been reported in relation to either patients presenting with non-carious cervical lesions (NCCLs) or as a result of data determined from laboratory (*in vitro*) investigations into this subject area. These findings include:

- the presence of such lesions amongst patients who seldom brush their teeth[2]
- the location of certain lesions, sometimes in subgingival areas where the action of wear produced by overzealous home care habits seems illogical as the location would not permit the brush to contact the affected area[14]
- where an isolated tooth may be affected (with adjacent teeth showing the absence of such lesions)[15]
- the reporting of NCCLs amongst animals,[14] as well as amongst prehistoric populations that existed prior to the popular use of toothbrushes[2]
- evidence from photo elastic studies and finite element analysis that showed the cervical region to be the zone of highest stress concentration[16]

- the presence of a negative correlation between tooth mobility and NCCLs, where a mobile tooth is likely to tilt and distribute stresses to the periodontal tissues and alveolar bone as opposed to the case of a stable tooth, which when loaded laterally will on the balance of probability flex in the cervical area, resulting in stress concentrations in the cervical (fulcrum) portion of the tooth[16]
- on the basis of the anecdotal observation of the authors, once these 'abrasive' lesions are restored and are retained, it is uncommon to observe the Class V type pattern developing on the restoration itself.

Clearly, there is an indication for further study into this controversial subject area. For the phenomenon of cervical TW, there seems to be consensus on using the term NCCL for these defects and acceptance that, as is the case with other types of TW, probably the wear causing NCCLs is multifactorial and is related to intrinsic and extrinsic mechanical factors as well as chemical factors. Figure 2.4 shows a patient with NCCLs on the buccal surfaces of the upper central incisors.

2.5 Chemical Wear

It would appear that TW by the process of *erosion* (often referred to as *erosive tooth wear*, ETW) has received far more focus than wear caused by any of the other primary mechanisms. Indeed, as noted above, there is evidence to suggest the involvement of the mechanism of erosion as a primary cause of TW amongst approximately nine-tenths of all patients presenting with clinical signs.[11]

Erosion (sometimes also referred to as *corrosion*) has been defined as 'a chemical–mechanical process resulting in the cumulative loss of dental hard tissues not caused by bacteria.'[17] ETW is therefore a multifactorial process, with acid being the main cause.[17]

It has been suggested that the acids that lead to tooth erosion are more potent than those involved as part of the pathogenesis of dental caries, with typical pH values of 5–1.2 that act over relatively shorter periods of time (15–60 seconds, as opposed to those involved with cariogenesis that are thought to act over time periods of 15–20 minutes).[1] Consequently, it has been postulated that erosive demineralisation is a much faster acting process than the acidic damage that takes place during the formation of a carious lesion, and typically results in little subsurface deterioration.[1] However, chronic exposure to acids is usually required to produce the TW lesions often seen clinically.[9]

Acidic substrates involved with dental erosion may have either:

- an *intrinsic* (or endogenous) source, namely gastric acid, or
- an *extrinsic* (exogenous) source, such as dietary, drinking habits, environmental or occupational acids.

The erosive patterns observed clinically will undoubtedly vary not only according to the source of the acid, but will also be influenced by the frequency and duration of exposure, the pH of the acid, and of course the buffering capacity offered. Hence, the patterns of wear observed can sometimes prove helpful in establishing a likely cause. However, it should also be noted that amongst cases with long-term acid exposure, the pattern of ETW in the oral cavity will most likely affect all surfaces, thereby rendering it challenging (if not indeed impossible) to determine the initial cause without a thorough patient history.[1]

Whilst the likely patterns stemming from a particular cause have been appraised below, in general TW lesions due to erosive mechanisms initially tend to demonstrate the presence of a glazed (sometimes described as a 'silky') appearance, with the loss of micro-anatomical enamel features (such as the perikymata) and the gradual development of a shallow, smooth surface.[1] Indeed, the latter appearance (together with the absence of any notable plaque deposits) is commonly viewed as an indicator of *active erosion*, whilst in contrast the presence of a stained surface may be suggestive of quiescence (based on the premise of an erosive factor not having sufficient contact time to remove dietary chromogens). At this stage, the presence of an intact rim of enamel tissue around the gingival margin (commonly referred to as the *gingival cuff*) can usually be seen; its presence is likely to be due to the neutralisation of acid by the gingival crevicular fluid.

With progression, the erosive lesion will typically show the loss of tooth contour with the concomitant flattening of the labial/buccal emergence profile (eventually leading to a concave profile). The loss of developmental ridges can also be seen to occur at this stage; macroscopically, it is not uncommon to see bilateral concave defects without the chalkiness or roughness of the affected surfaces.[9]

As the exposure of the dentine layer becomes more noticeable, the appearance of *cupping* of the occlusal surfaces begins to often take place, with enamel ridges surrounding the crater-like defect. However, the development of an occlusal cupping will not only occur due to erosive challenges, as mechanical factors are also necessary for this clinical presentation. Again, this emphasises that TW is almost always multifactorial in origin. The lesion may now take on a rather dulled appearance, but existing restorations may remain proud of the occluding surface. The latter can often provide a clue to help differentiate wear by erosive mechanisms as opposed to by attritional means. An analogous pattern of *grooving* may also be seen on the incisal edges of the anterior dentition, with scooped out depressions forming on the labial surfaces (often associated with extrinsic erosion).[1,9] At this stage, dentine hypersensitivity may be reported as a presenting complaint, especially amongst cases of active erosion, where acidic exposure will lead to the removal of the smear layer, followed by the opening of the dentinal tubules. Especially in younger people even a small cup can cause severe pain as the dentinal tubules are still wide open.

In the more advanced stages, ETW may manifest with the loss of the entire occlusal morphology, associated with the presence of a hollowed out occlusal surface and the appearances of concave depressions on the palatal surfaces of the maxillary anterior teeth.[9,17]

2.5.1 Intrinsic Chemical Wear

As stated above, the stomach is the source of intrinsic acid (with pH values of between 1 and 3), thus the regurgitation of the stomach contents which will lead to ETW. However, according to the consensus report of the European Federation of Conservative Dentistry in 2015, frequent regurgitation coupled with an extended period of activity is required for the impact to lead to significant tooth tissue loss; in contrast, infrequent activity (e.g. from occasional stomach disorders or morning sickness during pregnancy) is unlikely to be cause for real concern.[17]

However, there are a number of established medical conditions which can lead to ETW, including the following:[1,17]

a) *Gastro-oesophageal reflux disease (GORD/GERD)*: This condition is characterised by the involuntary passing of gastric contents into the oesophagus and
results from the laxity of the oesophageal sphincter. It is clinically sometimes
recognised by symptom of *heartburn* (burning retrosternal discomfort), but
this is not always a consistent feature, with many patient having no symptoms, commonly referred to as *silent GORD*. Other symptoms may include
regurgitation, dysphagia, non-cardiac chest pain, chronic cough, laryngeal
swelling, and chronic hoarseness.

   GORD may be associated with sphincter incompetence, increased gastric
pressure or increased gastric volume, and be a clinical sign amongst patients
suffering with conditions such as cerebral palsy, bronchitis, and hiatus hernia.
Associations have also been made with the diagnosis of GORD amongst
middle-aged men who may also be suffering with sleep apnoea and bruxism.
TW lesions due to GORD tend to manifest on the palatal surfaces of the
maxillary posterior teeth, as the refluxate typically displays a tendency to rise
towards the back of the throat and soft palate, as well as occlusal surfaces of
lower molar and premolar teeth, with cheeks and tongue protecting the
buccal and lingual surfaces of those teeth.[1]

b) *Regurgitation* of the gastric contents in the oral cavity. Regurgitation has been
linked with certain forms of gastrointestinal pathology, such as obstipation,
hiatal hernia, duodenal, and peptic ulceration.

c) *Rumination*: This is a voluntary habit that, although rare in Western society,
is associated with some cultures, as well as in bulimics, infants, and occasionally amongst individuals with learning disabilities and psychological illness,
such as depression. During rumination, the lower oesophageal sphincter is
relaxed, thus permitting recently swallowed foodstuff to be re-chewed and
swallowed again. The erosive pattern has been described to more likely be of
a generalised nature but may further involve the occlusal surfaces.[1]

d) *Eating disorders* that have been linked to TW include anorexia nervosa (AN)
and bulimia nervosa (BN) – both of which are characterised by the persistent
avoidance of food or a behaviour that impairs physical or psychosocial function, and are not related to any other medical condition; sufferers turn to food
and eating to express their psychological and emotional difficulties. Patients
with AN abstain from eating and vomiting may also be present occasionally.
However, AN patients often exhibit other typical factors associated with a
higher risk for TW such as hyposalivation and bruxism. Binge eating is associated with BN followed by behaviour to avoid weight gain with frequent bouts
of self-induced acts of vomiting. Cases of BM have been reported to occur in
1–3% of the female population (but not exclusively affecting young female
patients, with a male to female ratio of about 1:10), with sufferers attempting
to embrace the concepts of the 'ideal' body image associated with thinness.[18]

During the act of vomiting, the palatal surfaces of the maxillary teeth are most likely to be affected, as the tongue usually covers the mandibular teeth during the act of vomiting. As such, eating disorders and GORD may show identical clinical symptoms. However, immediately following the event, the combined actions of gravity, and cheek and lip movements during the act of swallowing will help distribute the vomitus residue to other areas of the mouth (inclusive of the lower jaw), thus with time it is probable that many (if not most) of the other teeth will also become involved.[1]

e) *Chronic alcoholism/alcohol induced gastritis*: Excessive alcoholic beverage consumption may lead to ETW by means of extrinsic wear, with some commonly consumed drinks such as red wine having relatively low reported pH values, such as 3.4.[1] This, coupled with the potential of intrinsic chemical wear associated with the habit of vomiting during periods of copious consumption, will exacerbate the risks of developing ETW with such habits. Figure 2.5 shows a patient with generalised intrinsic chemical TW.

2.5.2 Extrinsic Chemical Wear

Extrinsic factors may also have an important role in the pathogenesis of ETW. In Chapter 1, the impact of carbonated drinks (containing acids) in the aetiology of wear by erosion was briefly eluded to, and a list of the typical pH values and type of acid of some commonly consumed beverages provided. Additional food items of note that may be associated with extrinsic erosion include fruits (especially those containing citric or malic acid), pickles (and other foods containing vinegar, acetic acid), herbal tea, and spicy foods. Indeed, a study published by Ghai and Burke showed that certain components of Indian cooking, such as tomatoes and red chilli powder, have an erosive potential, with all basic masalas made and tested as part of their investigation showing a pH of less than 4.5.[19] The copious consumption of spicy foods may also lead to the provocation of GORD.[20] The frequent consumption of salad dressings has also been implicated as a potential causative factor for ETW, whilst it is also likely on the basis of the latter that a vegetarian diet would be associated with a higher occurrence of erosive defects.

Clearly, the risks of developing ETW will be heightened amongst patients who consume erosive food and drinks in greater quantities and with greater frequency. Furthermore, the method and pattern of consumption has been described as being relevant to the extent of ETW. Swallowing larger gulps over a shorter period of time may be less harmful than a habit comprising the processes of sipping and/or retention and/or swishing of the acidic drink prior to swallowing. Therefore the presentation of TW will mostly depend on the technique of swallowing and drinking/sipping.

However, the precise mechanism by which the substrate is consumed will also markedly affect the location where the wear lesion is most likely to develop. For instance, the act of drinking directly from a bottle, or allowing acidic drink to spill out when pulling out a straw, or the sucking of citrus fruits is likely to lead to labial/facial surface wear whilst the swishing of an acidic beverage prior to swallowing is more likely to be associated with widespread erosive wear affecting multiple posterior tooth surfaces.[1]

The consumption and/or use of certain medications, oral hygiene products, recreational drugs and dietary supplements has also been associated with an increased risk of developing ETW. Such compounds may include not only erosive substances but also agents that by the process of reducing the rate of salivary flow will lead to more bruxism can enhance the risk of ETW form direct factors. Provided below is a list of such substances:[11,17]

- acidic saliva stimulants
- low=pH mouthwashes
- iron tablets
- Bricanyl powder (used for the treatment of asthma)
- the drug Ecstasy
- preparations containing acetylsalicylic acid (such as aspirin)
- vitamin C (L-ascorbic acid) tablets when consumed in a chewable tablet form or used to prepare an effervescent drink.

Additionally, there are a number of drugs with associated unwanted sides effects of nausea or vomiting that can also indirectly be the cause of ETW. Examples of these drugs include oestrogens, opiates, tetracycline, levodopa, aminophylline, digitalis, and disulfiram.[9]

There are also some occupations where workers may become inadvertently exposed to acidic liquids or vapours that may lead to rapid ETW. However, it should be noted that this is a less common cause of ETW.[17] Examples of such occupations at higher risk for ETW include wine tasters, gas workers, those involved with metal plating (because of the use of various acids such as chromic, nitric, hydrofluoric and phosphoric acid), the galvanising industry (hydrochloric and sulphuric acid), and battery manufacturers (sulphuric acid). Due to modern guidelines for working environments, it is not likely these days that ETW is caused by the working space.

Regular swimming has also been linked with an increased risk of ETW amongst competitive swimmers, where by approximately 40% of a sample training in a pool of pH 2.7 showed signs of ETW.[21] The use of chlorinated gas and sodium hypochlorite to carry out pool disinfection, however, in the EU nowadays follows guidelines for swimming pools that recommend the pH to be between 7.2 and 8.0, which makes it unlikely that swimming pools play any role in the aetiology of tooth erosion.[22]

However, an indirect relation may exist between athletes and ETW, which is probably related to dehydration occurring during sport participation and the frequent intake of acidic sports drinks. This combines with cofactors such as clenching. It should be kept in mind that sports drinks and occupation can be for some patients a cofactor in the development of or increase in dental erosion. However, it is unlikely that one or two isolated factors will be responsible for this multifactorial condition.

In relation to the clinical appearance of lesions caused by ETW involving extrinsic factors, lesions occurring on the labial surfaces of maxillary anterior teeth typically tend to take the form of scooped-out depressions, whilst lesions initiated by intrinsic acid sources are most often seen on the palatal surfaces of the maxillary anterior teeth, resulting in a concave depression of the entire palatal surface.[1] The term *perimolysis* has been used to describe the classical lesions seen as a result of chronic vomiting, localised to the palatal surfaces of the maxillary anterior teeth. The presence of active caries lesions in the area with erosive wear may implicate the (over)use of sugar-containing low-pH drinks and food.

Figure 2.6 shows an example of extrinsic chemical wear.

2.6   Cofactors

There are a number of factors (often referred to as cofactors), which although they are not directly responsible for the pathogenesis of TW, their presence in conjunction with the primary mechanisms described above can exacerbate the rate of progression. Many relate to the rate of salivary flow and/or the quality of the saliva produced.

Saliva has a well-established role for the protection of the dental hard tissues against TW by offering the following important functions:[10]

- buffering
- dilution of the acidic substances[17]
- acid clearance
- hard tissue remineralisation, by providing calcium, phosphate and fluoride ions to eroded enamel and dentine
- lubrication and the formation of the acquired pellicle.

It is therefore unsurprising to see signs of TW amongst patients suffering with *xerostomia* (the sensation of dry mouth) or with varying degree of hyposalivation. Salivary flow rates can be reduced by a number of factors, including high levels of exercise, systemic disease such as Sjogrens syndrome, or taking some prescription medication, such as antidepressive and antihypertensive drugs.[17]

Additionally, amongst patients with hard tissue defects such as hypominerilsation or hereditary dysplasias such as amelogensis imperfecta, which affect the enamel tissues as well as the extent of calcification with the tissues, TW is more likely to occur as such teeth will be more susceptible to wear by erosion.[20]

2.7   Conclusion

It is not always possible to determine the precise causes of TW, especially given the multitude of factors that have the potential to cause this condition and the likelihood of them (in some cases, such as dietary acid or inappropriate toothbrushing habits) being frequently encountered by many patients.

However, in order to effectively treat a patient with signs of TW, it is imperative to properly manage the underlying cause. Knowledge of the primary mechanisms (intrinsic and extrinsic mechanical and chemical factors) that are associated with TW as well as some of the common causes, the taking of a clear and accurate patient history, as well as attention to the presenting clinical features may prove vital in attaining a successful outcome with such patients when seeking to provide care.

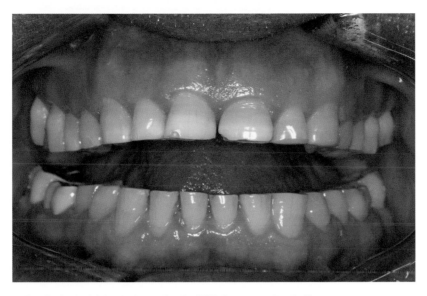

Figure 2.1 Patient with intrinsic mechanical TW due to tooth grinding.

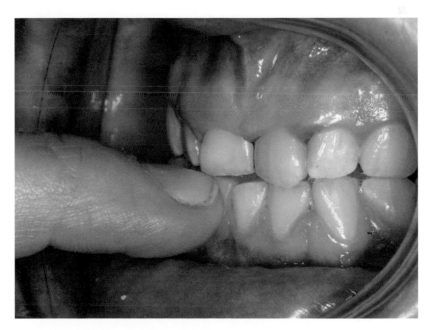

Figure 2.2 Extrinsic mechanical TW from a patient with a nail-biting habit.

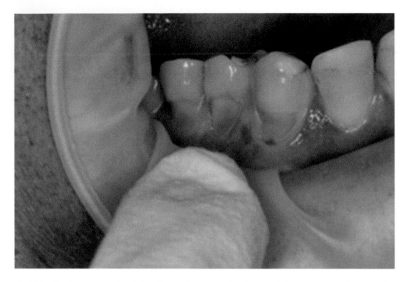

Figure 2.3 Extrinsic mechanical TW shown here on the lower right canine and premolar teeth due to excessive and incorrect toothbrushing technique.

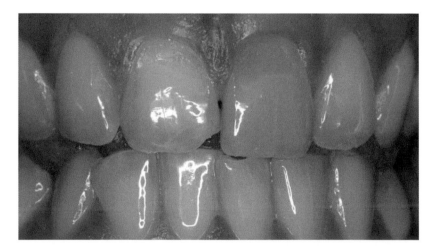

Figure 2.4 Patient with NCCLs on the buccal aspect of the upper central incisors.

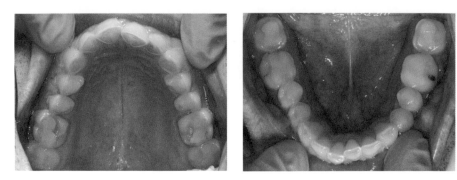

Figure 2.5 Views of the upper and lower dentition of a patient with intrinsic chemical TW due to acid reflux.

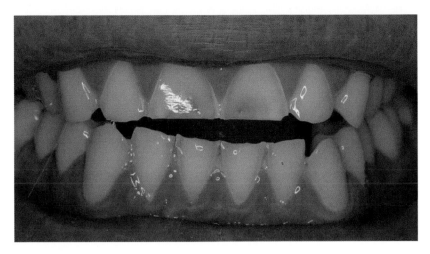

Figure 2.6 Extrinsic chemical TW on the upper and lower incisors (notably on the central incisors) due to excessive citrus fruit consumption.

References

1 Kaladonis, J. (2012). Oral diagnosis and treatment planning: Part 4. Non-carious tooth surface loss and assessment of risk. *Br. Dent. J.* 213: 155–161.
2 Johansson, A., Johansson, A.K., Omar, R., and Carlsson, G. (2008). Rehabilitation of the worn dentition. *J. Oral Rehabil.* 35: 548–566.
3 Loomans, B., Opdam, N., Attin, T. et al. (2017). Severe tooth wear: European consensus statement on management guidelines. *J. Adhes. Dent.* 19: 111–119.
4 Locker, D. (1988). Measuring oral health: a conceptual framework. *Community Dent. Health* 5 (1): 3–18.
5 Slade, G. and Spencer, A. (1994). Development and evaluation of the oral health impact profile. *Community Dent. Health* 11: 3–11.
6 Sterenborg, B.A.M.M., Bronkhorst, E.M., Wetselaar, P. et al. (2018 Feb 3). The influence of management of tooth wear on oral health-related quality of life. *Clin. Oral Investig.* https://doi.org/10.1007/s00784-018-2355-8.
7 Larsson, P., John, M.T., Nilner, K. et al. (2010). Development of an orofacial esthetic scale in prosthodontic patients. *Int. J. Prosthodont.* 23 (3): 249–256.
8 Larsson, P., John, M.T., Nilner, K., and List, T. (2010). Reliability and validity of the orofacial esthetic scale in prosthodontic patients. *Int. J. Prosthodont.* 23 (3): 257–262.
9 Hattab, F. and Yassin, O. (2000). Etiology and diagnosis of tooth wear: a literature review and presentation of selected cases. *Int. J. Prosthodont.* 13: 101–107.
10 Yule, P. and Barclay, S. (2015). Worn dentition by toothwear? Aetiology, diagnosis and management revisited. *Dent. Update* 42: 525–532.
11 Smith, B. and Knight, J. (1984). A comparison of patterns of tooth wear with aetiological factors. *Br. Dent. J.* 157: 16–19.
12 Watson, M. and Burke, F. (2000). Investigation and treatment of patients with teeth affected by tooth substance loss: a review. *Dent. Update* 27: 175–183.

13 Litonuja, L., Andreana, S., Bush, P., and Cohen, R. (2003). Tooth wear: attrition, erosion and abrasion. *Quintessence Int.* 34: 435–446.

14 Milosevic, A. (1998). Toothwear: aetiology and presentation. *Dent. Update* 25: 6–11.

15 Imfeld, T. (1996). Dental erosion. Definition, classification and links. *Eur. J. Oral Sci.* 104: 151–155.

16 Grippo J, S.M. and Coleman, T. (2012). Abfraction, abrasion, biocorrosion, and the enigma of noncarious cervical lesions: a 20-year prespective. *J. Esthet. Restor. Dent.* 24: 10–23.

17 Carvalho, T., Colon, P., Ganss, C. et al. (2016). Consensus report of the European federation of conservative dentistry: erosive tooth wear – diagnosis and management. *Swiss Dent. J.* 126: 342–346.

18 Kelleher, M., Bomfim, D., and Austin, R. (2012). Biologically based restorative management of tooth wear. *Int. J. Dent.* 2012: 1–9.

19 Ghai, N. and Burke, F. (2012). Mouthwatering but erosive? A preliminary assessment of the acidity of basic sauce used in many Indian dishes. *Dent. Update* 39: 721–726.

20 Bartlett, D., Evans, D., and Snith, B. (1997). Oral regurgitation after reflux provoking meals: a possible cause of dental erosion? *J. Oral Rehabil.* 24: 102–108.

21 Centrewall, B., Armstron, C., Funkhouser, L., and Elzay, R. (1986). Erosion of dental enamel among competitive swimmers at a gas-chlorinated swimming pool. *Am. J. Epidemiol.* 123: 641–647.

22 Kontaxopoulou, I. and Alam, S. (2015). Risk assessment for tooth wear. *Prim. Dent. J.* 4 (2): 25–29.

Further Reading

Gandara, B.K. and Truelove, E.L. (1999). Diagnosis and management of dental erosion. *J. Contemp. Dent. Pract.* 1: 16–23. Review.

Ganss, C. and Lussi, A. (2014). Diagnosis of erosive tooth wear. *Monogr. Oral Sci.* 25: 22–31.

Lussi, A. and Ganss, C. (2014). *Erosive Tooth Wear for Diagnosis to Therapy*, Monographs in Oral Science, vol. 25. Karger.

Romeed, S., Malik, R., and Dunne, S. Stress Analysis of Occlusal Forces in Canine Teeth and Their Rolein the Development of Non-Carious Cervical Lesions: Abfraction. *International Journal of Dentistry* 2012: 234845.

3

The Clinical Assessment and Diagnosis of the Wear Patient

3.1 Introduction

The foundation for successful treatment planning in dentistry is to a large extent dependent on the ability of the treating clinician to attain an accurate and contemporaneous patient history, as well as carry out a meticulous clinical examination (whilst also preparing and keeping appropriate patient records). Treatment planning should, in general, aim to fulfil the patient's realistic expectations, provide an outcome that boasts functional and aesthetic success (spanning beyond the short term), and, where possible, utilise techniques that involve minimal intervention.[1]

In previous chapters, the typical macro- and microscopic features associated with the exposure of dental hard tissues to the primary aetiological mechanisms responsible for the pathogenesis of tooth wear (TW) have been described. This chapter will focus on the clinical assessments and evaluations that should be performed when a patient attends for a dental examination, with emphasis placed on those aspects that are more pertinent to a wearing dentition to help establish a diagnosis/diagnoses and ultimately determine a logical plan for future care. Such plans, when of a biologically prudent variety,[2] should aim to consider:

- the preservation of the residual tooth tissue
- the pragmatic enhancement of the existing aesthetic presentation
- the restoration of patient confidence (in relation to self-directed care as well as to optimally conserving the residual tooth tissue for as long as possible)
- the restoration of function
- the provisions for failure.

As part of the assessment protocol, it is also important to identify any potential *physical*, *social*, and/or *medical markers* that may indicate a higher risk for the occurrence of unnecessary tooth tissue loss,[3] thereby enabling the prescription of an appropriate course of care, as well as making a concerted effort to determine all of the likely causes. A general description of the aforementioned markers is provided below, with a brief note on risk assessments.

When carrying out patient assessments many clinicians adopt the use of information gathering templates. These have the clear merit of steering the clinician towards an overall systematic approach, as well as helping to avoid key omissions

Practical Procedures in the Management of Tooth Wear, First Edition. Subir Banerji, Shamir Mehta, Niek Opdam and Bas Loomans.
© 2020 John Wiley & Sons Ltd. Published 2020 by John Wiley & Sons Ltd.
Companion website: www.wiley.com/go/banerji/toothwear

which may prove to be of diagnostic significance. As part of the account provided below, portions of an assessment template (based on one used for generic prosthodontic purposes) used by the authors have been ascribed to each section. This may prove of practical assistance to the reader when designing an analogous protocol to meet their specific needs.

3.2 The Initial Assessment: The Presenting Complaint and the History of the Presenting Complaint

The initial patient assessment should optimally take place in a relaxed setting and permit the patient to voice their views. Emphasis should be placed on actively *listening* to the patient's concerns and attitudes.

In the first instance, it is of course appropriate to attain and record essential patient data (name, gender, date of birth, address, and contact and medical correspondence details). The completion of a pre-treatment evaluation document can prove helpful.

The accuracy and importance of the chief complaint must be evaluated. According to Loomans et al.[4] the reasons for a patient to seek help (with a likely diagnosis of pathological TW) may include the following:

1) *Sensitivity and/or pain*: Dentinal hypersensitivity may be reported amongst cases displaying dentine exposure where the rate of tissue loss is likely to exceed the reparative capacity of the dentinal-pulp complex with the concomitant absence of the smear layer. Where hard tissue loss may be excessive, the progressive loss of dentine tissue may culminate in the patient experiencing dental pain, pulpal inflammation, necrosis and/or periapical pathology.[5] Indeed, a prevalence rate for undiagnosed apical pathology of 12.7% was reported by Wazani et al. amongst a sample of patients attending a UK dental hospital suffering with TW;[6] analogous rates have been reported by other groups.[7] The actual rates of apical pathology amongst TW patients are likely to relate to the severity of the wear pattern present.

   Some patients with TW may also report a history of soft tissue trauma/irritation due to the progressive sharpening of their teeth, whilst others may also describe the presence of possible symptoms of temporomandibular disorder(s) (TMDs) that may be associated with the presence of TW by intrinsic mechanical means, e.g. attrition. However, the relationship between TMD and the presence of wear ascribed primarily to attrition is by no means consistent.

2) *Impaired orofacial aesthetics* (due to the loss of dental hard tissue resulting in fractured, discoloured or shortened clinical crowns/restorations or a reduced occlusal vertical dimension, OVD).

3) *Difficulties with chewing and eating*: Severe TW may sometimes lead to a complete loss of the occlusal anatomy, which might hamper the chewing efficacy.

4) *'Crumbling' of the dental hard tissues and/or restorations*, threatening the integrity of their teeth.

5) *General concerns about the condition and longevity of their teeth*, where the presence of TW may have been identified at the conclusion of the appointment or following a previous course of care.

It is interesting to note the outcomes of a review of the clinical records of 290 patients referred to the Liverpool University Dental Hospital, UK.[6] These determined the most common presenting complaints from patients suffering with TW to be related to:

- aesthetics (59%)
- sensitivity (40%)
- functional problems (17%)
- pain (14%).

Having noted the existence of a complaint, it is important to gain a full history of the nature and duration of the symptoms/complaint.

However, based on anecdotal clinical observations, it is by no means uncommon for a patient with TW (inclusive of cases with severe tooth tissue loss) to *not express any concerns* (at least when initially verbally quizzed, especially amongst cases displaying a slowly progressive pattern of TW) where the condition may indeed have become one of an 'acceptable' nature to the patient. The use of a pre-examination questionnaire template may be helpful to obtain a view on the level of oral health-related quality of life (OHRQoL) and the orofacial appearance of patients. A validated questionnaire on OHRQoL is the *Oral Health Impact Profile (OHIP)* and this may prove beneficial under such circumstances to gain an insight into how the presence of possible TW may be impacting on their quality of life.[8] The OHIP is the most frequently used oral-specific measure for OHRQoL. It is a questionnaire that contains 49 statements organised in seven domains: functional limitation, physical pain, psychological discomfort, physical disability, psychological disability, social disability, and handicap.[8]

With the use of a shortened version of the OHIP (OHIP-14), Li and Bernabe[9] showed that adults with severe wear reported higher domain scores with the categories of experiencing *psychological discomfort* and *psychological disability* (such as feeling self-conscious or tense, difficulty relaxing or embarrassment), with feelings likely to have been triggered by poor appearance (especially when involving the aesthetic zone), dentine hypersensitivity as well as the motivation to seek care.

3.3 Medical History

The attainment of an accurate and contemporaneous medical history is mandatory. Many practitioners opt to use a template medical history form to assist with this process. It is beyond the scope of this text to discuss the relevance of the medical history and its impact on the provision of dental care. However, in brief, the patient's medical history (and status) may:

- preclude them from attending necessary lengthy or frequent treatment sessions
- require a modification of the treatment protocol

- may sometimes contraindicate certain types of treatment such as an allergy to a material or product
- the underlying medical condition itself may prove to be directly contributory towards the clinical diagnosis, perhaps in an indirect manner, via the taking of medication or supplements contribute towards the pathogenesis of TW.

Further to Chapter 2, some noteworthy medical conditions in this context include the following:[10]

- *Gastric disorders* such as gastro-oesophageal reflux (GORD), gastric ulceration, sphincter incompetence, hiatus hernia, rumination, regurgitation, oesophagitis, and increased gastric volume and pressure. In Chapter 2, some of the clinical signs and symptoms associated with conditions such as GORD are listed. It is perhaps also relevant to take note of patients who may be on prescription medication for this condition, such as *proton pump inhibitors* or *H₂ antagonists*, especially amongst patients who may not be able to offer an accurate and concise medical history. Table 3.1 provides a list of commonly used examples of such drugs.
- *Vomiting tendencies* that may arise as a result of psychosomatic, gastrointestinal, and/or metabolic conditions, or where nausea may occur as a side effect of medical treatments or drugs being prescribe for the management of another condition, or indeed morning sickness during pregnancy.
- *Eating disorders*, especially those associated with self-induced vomiting such as bulimia nervosa (BN) also referred to as '*ox hunger*', whereby questioning in relation to prior and current slimming habits, views of self-image, and knowledge of the patient's actual weight may prove helpful in attempting to reach a possible diagnosis.[10] Table 3.2 lists some of the key clinical features associated with BN.[11] The dental practitioner may indeed be the first person to suspect such a psychological disorder.
- *The taking of potentially erosive medication/supplements* such as hydrochloric acid for achlohydria (lack of gastric acid), iron preparations, and/or chewable vitamin C tablets, the possible use of asthma medication in the form of inhalational aerosols, which may act directly (or indirectly by leading to a possible relaxation of the oesophageal sphincter), and/or drugs that may act to inadvertently reduce the production of saliva, such as diuretics and antidepressants.
- *Conditions that may reduce saliva*, such as Sjogrens syndrome, Prader–Willi syndrome, and congenital rubella.[3]

Table 3.1 Commonly prescribed drugs used to treat GORD.

Proton pump inhibitor drugs	H₂ antagonist drugs
Omeprazole	Ranitidine
Esomeprazole	Famotidine
Pantoprazole	Cimetidine
Rabeprazole	

Table 3.2 The key features associated with bulimia nervosa.

Predominantly involves female patients in their early 20s (male to female ratio of approximately 1:10)

Patients often suffer with a perception of low self-image

Primarily involves subjects in industrialised Western societies

Tendency towards binge eating/purging; purging may be associated with metabolic disturbances and electrolyte imbalance

Normal body weight (until anorexia nervosa comes into contention)

Sufferers are often intelligent and have an inclination towards compulsive habits

Reported patterns of drug and alcohol abuse and self-mutilation

---

Source: Adapted from Moazzez and Bartlett.[11]

- *Psychological conditions* such as; anxiety,[12] attention deficit hyperactivity disorder (ADHD), inattention and/or hyperactivity-impulsivity, where the likelihood of demonstrating bruxism may be increased.[13]
- *Chronic alcoholism*, which may also be associated with regurgitation or reflux, as well as possible wear by attrition due to a tendency towards bruxism.[11]
- *A history of radiation therapy involving the head and neck region.*

3.4 Dental and Socio-behavioural History

The taking of an appropriate dental and socio-behavioural history is of paramount importance in the case of a patient presenting with TW as it may not only yield vital clues as to the possible aetiology but also help to provide appropriate care. Aspects to note include the following:[10]

- *Oral hygiene home care habits*: the method and frequency of tooth brushing (especially noting a relationship between the timing of brushing and eating, drinking or vomiting – which may exacerbate abrasive wear of a tooth softened by prior acid exposure, especially within the first hour), the relative dentine abrasivity of the dentifrice used, the filament arrangement, density, and texture of toothbrush used,[14] a history of the use of any mouthwash agents, and the use of any topical fluorides.
- *Diet history*, noting the patterns of acidic food and beverage consumption as well as the actual methods of consumption (swishing erosive drinks, retaining erosive agents prior to swallowing and/or the use of a straw) and the presence of a vegetarian diet. Some patients may also demonstrate the habit of holding citrus fruits against their teeth. The role of spicy foods in erosive wear is discussed in Chapter 2.

    The process of conducting a *diet analysis* involving recording the intake of *all* food and drinks over a period of three days (*three-day diet diary*) may prove highly valuable.[10] The importance of recording data in the prescribed manner, ensuring accuracy, is essential to a successful outcome with this process. When asking patients to fill in a diet diary, one should be aware of the risk of attaining 'socially desirable' answers.

- *Alcohol intake* (as discussed above) as well as any habits of smoking and caffeine intake, which have been reported to aggravate bruxism.[12]
- *Psychological stress levels, sleep apnoea and a habit of snoring*, which may also serve to aggravate a bruxist tendency.[12]
- *Recreational factors*, such as vigorous exercise (which may result in dehydration, especially if erosive 'sports drinks' are consumed post exercise), wine tasting, and the taking of recreational drugs such as Ecstasy, which is associated with reduced saliva and excessive clenching, often manifesting as occlusal attrition (as opposed to incisal attrition).
- *Occupational related factors*, which, as discussed in Chapter 2 may include environmental acid exposure and/or abrasive wear seen amongst carpenters, musicians, and hairdressers stemming from the use of their teeth to hold nails, mouthpieces, and hair clips, respectively.

At this stage, it is also relevant to determine the patient's previous dental experiences, including any difficulties that may have been encountered, to ascertain their level of unease, apprehension, and anxiety of dentistry as well as to appraise their expectations at an early stage. Dental phobic patients and patients who lack the motivation to maintain a high standard of oral hygiene may be more suited to relatively simple, low-maintenance, minimally invasive forms of treatment. Patients with unrealistic expectations or patients without any demand for treatment may require further counselling, especially prior to embarking upon complex, irreversible forms of dental treatment to improve their commitment to a possible restorative treatment.[1]

Knowledge of each of the above factors will undoubtedly help to tailor an appropriate plan of care, but even knowing all these factors, it is sometimes not possible to find the main aetiological factors causing the TW.

Figure 3.1 provides a summary of the key features of the assessment protocol used when gathering relevant patient history. For the collection of a medical history, a separate template is usually used.

3.5   Patient Examination

3.5.1   The Extra-oral Examination

The extra-oral appraisal should include an assessment of the:

- temporomandibular joints (TMJs) and associated musculature
- cervical lymph nodes and salivary glands
- facial (and dento-facial) features such as facial proportions, symmetry, facial shape, profile and width, and lip morphology and mobility.

The process of undertaking a TMJ and muscle examination[15] should aim to assess and record the following:

- *The range of movement*: The degree of maximum mandibular opening should be determined by measuring the inter-incisal distance: any distance less than 35 mm is considered to be restricted. The degree of maximum movements on the undertaking of lateral movements should also be determined; the normal is accepted to be about 12 mm. A note of the presence of any mandibular deviation on opening and closure movements is advised.

- The presence of any *TMJ tenderness* initiated by the palpation of features in the pre-auricular region, by palpation involving the placement of the index fingers into the external auditory meati and asking the patient to open and close, and by attempting to gently manipulate the mandible into a retruded position.
- The detection of any anomalous *joint sounds* (ideally with the aid of a stethoscope). It is appropriate to note the presence of a 'click', and if it occurs determine whether it is associated with the symptom of pain, the presence of a single or multiple clicks, and the point of the opening/closure cycle at which the click is heard (early or late). Variations may help to determine a likely diagnosis. The presence of *dislocation* or *crepitation sounds* should also be noted.
- The muscular examination should involve the bilateral palpitation of the masticatory muscles. This is performed by pressing the muscles between the thumb placed extra-orally and index finger intra-orally whilst concomitantly noting the presence of hypertrophy, tenderness or discomfort, particularly in areas of muscle insertion. The anterior and posterior temporalis muscles and the superficial and deep masseter muscles are perhaps the most relevant in this context. Masseteric hypertrophy has been associated with the pattern of wear by intrinsic mechanical wear. Also note a possible asymmetric representation of the most important chewing muscles (masseter and temporalis), which may be related to abnormal (dental) habits.

Examination of the salivary glands should include bilateral palpation of the parotid and submandibular salivary; in health, these glands should not be palpable. The (non-tender) enlargement of the parotid glands has been described to occur amongst patients with alcoholism, diabetes, Sjogren's syndrome, eating disorders (such as BN), and HIV infection as well as a variety of malignant/non-malignant states.

The role of hyposalivation as a co-factor for the pathogenesis of the wear lesion is eluded to in Chapter 2. Patients suffering with hyposalivation may complain of difficulty with:[16]

- swallowing, especially dry foods
- controlling their dentures
- phonation, as the tongue tends to stick to the palate.

Patients may also complain of unpleasant taste or loss of sense of taste, or halitosis.

The *facial features* which should be assessed as part of the extra-oral examination include:[17]

- the vertical facial proportions
- facial symmetry
- facial profile
- facial shape and width.

The human face when observed from a frontal direction can be divided into three zones: the *upper third*, which includes the area between the hairline and the ophriac line (brow line), the *middle third*, which ranges from the ophriac line to the interalar line (base of the nose), and the *lower third*, which includes the area between the interalar line and the tip of the chin.[17]

The lower third region appears to be the most significant in determining the overall facial appearance and is the zone over which the dental operator has the most control. It may also become adversely affected in the presence of a severely worn dentition.[17] The term OVD refers to the vertical distance between two selected anatomical points when the maxillary teeth are occluding with the mandibular teeth. Hence, the loss of tooth tissue may culminate in the loss of OVD, which may impact upon the lower third region, with some patients displaying an *overclosed* appearance, and also may also affect patient function, comfort, and aesthetics.[18]

The exact amount of loss of OVD is difficult to determine as not only the loss of tooth material, but also an amount of compensatory alveolar growth has occurred. It is relatively easy to make an assumption of the first aspect, but the exact amount of compensatory growth is almost impossible to determine. The best way to make an assumption is to compare the distance of the lower third of the face with the middle and upper third of the face.

It is therefore appropriate to determine the magnitude of OVD loss at this stage. In some patients the loss of OVD may lead to an increased *freeway space* (FWS), but in the majority of patients this cannot be seen due to compensatory growth.

Measurement of the FWS can be accomplished with the use of a set of callipers or a Willis gauge. It has been suggested that the physiological FWS should be approximately 2–4 mm. It should be noted however, that the latter methods are by no means highly accurate.[18] Other techniques that can be used for the evaluation of FWS include the use of phonetic assessments (particularly sibilant sounds), facial soft tissue contour analysis, jaw tracking, and electrical muscle stimulation techniques.[19] However, all of these techniques seems to be of limited value. Figure 3.2 provides a summary of the extra-oral findings that are likely to be appraised and recorded during this part of the examination process.

Figure 3.3 illustrates a case of severe tooth wear with and without compensatory growth.

When considering *facial symmetry*, the facial midline (the imaginary line connecting the nasion to the base of the philtrum) and the interpupillary line are the most commonly utilised *vertical and horizontal reference planes*, respectively. Aesthetic harmony is said to be attained where the vertical and horizontal reference planes are perpendicular to each other, and the dental midline is co-incident with the facial midline.[17]

The interpupillary line provides the operator with a key reference axis in determining the ultimate position of the incisal, gingival, and occlusal planes, respectively. This may prove highly relevant in a patient displaying anterior tooth wear in helping to plan restorative rehabilitation. However, caution needs to be exercised where the interpupillary line may be canted; under such circumstances, the horizon is perhaps better applied as the horizontal reference plane.

The *lateral facial profile* is most appropriately assessed with the patient adopting a natural head posture. Three forms of facial profile have been described in the contemporary literature:

- normal profile
- convex profile
- concave profile.

The *E-line* (formed by connecting the tip of the nose to the tip of the chin) is also frequently applied to determine facial profile. A normal profile is thought to exist when the upper and lower lips are 4 and 2 mm, respectively, posterior to the E-line, but it is necessary to accommodate racial and gender variations.

Classically, four types of basic *facial shape* have been described in the literature:

- ovoid
- square
- tapering
- square-tapering (Leon Williams classification).

This classification system has historically been used to determine appropriate moulds for removable denture prosthesis, albeit on a purely arbitrary basis. More recently, four typological categories have been described for particular facial shapes:[20]

- lymphatic (rounded full features with a timid personality)
- sanguine (prominent, thick, well-defined features associated with intransigence and spontaneity)
- nervous (large forehead, thin delicate features with an anxious disposition)
- bilious (rectangular and muscular features coupled with a dominant persona).

The application of such concepts to the worn dentition may help to plan the ultimate morphological outcome when planning the restorative rehabilitation of worn dentition involving the anterior teeth, where in some cases there may be little available clue to the original tooth form (such as archive close up photographs).

The lips should be analysed for their morphology and level of mobility, noting the width, fullness (thin, medium or thick), and symmetry of the lips.

Lip mobility describes the amount of lip movement that occurs when a patient smiles. The amount of anterior tooth display should be determined with the lips in a resting position and a dynamic position. The resting position of the lips has classically been used to determine the ultimate position of the incisal edges of the anterior maxillary teeth when undertaking complete denture prosthetics. Vig and Brundo[21] have determined the average ranges for tooth display at rest according to age:

- aged 30 years: 3.0–3.5 mm
- aged 50 years: 1.0–1.5 mm
- aged 70 years: 0.0–0.5 mm.

These values may serve as useful guidelines, particularly when contemplating the lengthening of the incisal edges using fixed prosthodontic means, as may be the case when managing a worn anterior dentition. Phonetic tests such as the enunciation of the 'F' and 'V' sounds can also be used to help verify the correct spatial relationship between the incisal edges of the anterior maxillary teeth and the lower lip, as discussed further in Chapter 8.

Visualisation: Clinical advice is to not only make a set of pictures (intra- and extra-oral), but also to make a short video of the patient. This, in combination with extra-oral pictures, can give a good impression of a patient at rest, and during speaking and laughing, and can give a good impression of the aesthetics and desired length of the incisors.

3.5.2   The Intra-oral Examination

In relation to a patient with TW, the intra-oral examination should include the undertaking and recording of:

- a soft tissue assessment
- an assessment of the dental hard tissues
- a periodontal examination
- an occlusal assessment
- an evaluation of the aesthetic zone
- an appraisal of any edentulous spaces.

Figure 3.4 provides a summary of the intra-oral features that would be recorded during the examination appointment(s), excluding details relating to the occlusal, aesthetic, and edentulous spaces.

3.5.2.1   The Soft Tissue Assessment

Additional soft tissue findings that may be of further relevance to the diagnosis and management of a patient with TW include the signs of buccal keratosis, scalloping of the tongue and cheek biting, which may indicate a habit suggestive of parafunctional tooth clenching and grinding habits, and signs of hyposalivation. The presence of the latter may be crudely indicated by the adherence of the mirror head to the mucosa surfaces. Amongst patients with dry mouth it is not uncommon to see signs of lipstick or food debris sticking to the teeth or soft tissues, thin lines of frothy saliva forming along lines of contact of the oral soft tissues, and/or a lack of salivary pooling in the floor of the mouth. The tongue may also appear dry, sometimes with a lobulated and erythematous presentation, with signs of the partial or complete loss of the papillae.[16] Saliva may not be expressible from the parotid ducts.

The use of the *Challacombe Scale*[22] may prove helpful in being able to clinically identify the presence of dry mouth, quantify the severity, and provide some guidance for the appropriate treatment options.

3.5.2.2   Assessment of the Dental Hard Tissues

Accurate examination of the dental hard tissues should be undertaken and charting completed to record the presence and absence of teeth, dental caries, sound and defective restorations, tooth fractures, cracks, wear of mechanical and chemical origin (intrinsic and extrinsic), and any tooth malformations. The extent and location of any caries should also be noted, as should the type and extent of all dental restorations. Dental restorations should be further assessed for their clinical acceptability. The presence of any secondary caries, open contacts, and other food traps and wear facets, present on either the remaining dental tissues or the functional surfaces, should also be noted and suitably documented. Besides this detailed information we need to assess the patient's risk factors, e.g. intense bruxism activity.

The use of a sharp probe is helpful as is the action of drying the hard tissues using air from a three-in-one syringe and using suitable magnification with illumination. It is helpful to ensure that the teeth are also stain and plaque free. The macroscopic features associated with the mechanisms that produce wear are described in Chapter 2. A good working knowledge of these features is highly appropriate.

Having ascertained the presence of TW, it is appropriate to also determine the pattern, extent and severity of wear, as well as noting the quality and quantity of the residual tooth tissues (inclusive of the presence of any defects that may result from hypomineralisation and/or hypocalcification of the hard tissues). For further details, including the common indices used in conjunction with this process, refer to Chapter 5.

3.5.2.3 Periodontal Assessments

The periodontal examination of a patient with TW should aim to accurately note:[23]

- their oral hygiene levels (commonly denoted as being good, moderate or poor)
- the presence of any colour and morphological anomalies of the gingivae
- bleeding on probing
- exudate or any halitosis
- the patient's home care.

Probing to determine *clinical attachment loss and to detect any sites with bleeding on probing* is the conventional method used to assess the presence of any gingival and periodontal pathology. In addition to the presence of any periodontal pocketing, it is also appropriate to determine the presence of any tooth mobility as well as the presence and extent of any gingival recession and furcation involvement(s).

In the UK, perhaps the most common starting point for all periodontal examinations is the *basic periodontal examination* (BPE). The outcomes obtained from this assessment may indicate the need for further periodontal investigation(s).

Restorative dental procedures should ideally be avoided in the presence of unstable oral health. For cases of tooth wear where restorative care is planned, it is also advisable to make note of the baseline *clinical attachment levels* (periodontal pocketing and recession), *plaque scores*, and *bleeding scores*.[24] Restorative procedures may not only prove more challenging to execute in the presence of gingival and periodontal instability, but the iatrogenic damage sustained by the supporting tissues when undertaking such procedures may exacerbate any periodontal concerns. Furthermore, longer-term periodontal breakdown may be accentuated by an alteration in local conditions which may encourage plaque stagnation and render good oral hygiene practice more challenging, such as those resulting from the provision of dental restorations, or by increasing the mechanical loading onto affected teeth (which may happen with a patient displaying parafunctional tendencies in relation to clenching or grinding habits or when the crown:root ratio is changed, as is sometimes the case when undertaking restorative rehabilitation), which may concomitantly result in further periodontal breakdown (*occlusal trauma*).[25]

Where periodontal surgery is being planned, it is again imperative to carry out appropriate periodontal assessments (such as clinical attachment levels and the gingival biotype) to avoid iatrogenic damage to the periodontal tissues (such as the invasion of the biological width and the associated consequences, including gingival recession), which may occur post-operatively.

3.5.2.4 The Occlusal Examination

Occlusion has been defined as 'an integral (but not necessarily central) part within the stomato-gnathic system (SGS) that relates teeth, not only to other teeth, but, importantly, to the other components of the SGS during normal function, parafunction and dysfunction'.[26] Accordingly, the stomato-gnathic system (SGS) includes the TMJ, muscles, periodontium, and other teeth.

In the presence of a wearing dentition (as well as following the processes of mesial drift, post-extraction tilt and drift, and the placement of restorations in either supra- or infra-occlusion), directly and/or as a result of the compensatory mechanisms that exist to maintain the functionality of the masticatory system (such as dento-alevolar compensation, as discussed further in Chapter 5), changes to the occlusal scheme may take place.

In order to attain longer-term success with restorative care it is paramount to develop a fundamental appreciation of the concepts of clinical occlusion. Failure to provide a mechanically sound masticatory system following the placement of dental restorations that is not conducive to optimal function concomitantly offering desirable levels of load distribution with minimal trauma to the investing structures will likely culminate in premature restorative failure. There is also a risk of causing iatrogenic damage to the residual tissues, as well as possible instability concerning the spatial position of a tooth or teeth within the dental arches.[25]

An assessment of the patient's occlusal scheme should be carried out with reference to this standard. The assessment should take into account both static and dynamic components of the patient's occlusal scheme. The features that should be appraised and recorded as part of this section of the dental examination are summarised in Figure 3.5. The *static occlusal examination* should take note of the presence of any of the following features:

- tooth rotations, tilting, drifting, supra-eruption
- crowding
- spacing

- overjet
- overbite (including open bites and cross bites)
- occlusal vertical dimension
- FWS.

The assessment of these features will help to establish the presence of any *malocclusions* and further categorise the *inter-arch occlusal relationships (such as incisor, canine* and *molar segment classifications)*. It is also important to establish the *loss of posterior support* at this stage, and determine whether or not this is a factor to consider in cases displaying further anterior tooth tissue loss.

The clinician must therefore be aware of the concepts of the ideal occlusal scheme. This is discussed further in Chapter 5. However, it must be stated that the exact role of occlusion in relation to TW has not been proven and is often based on traditional theories of occlusion.

The inter-cuspal position (ICP), also commonly referred to as the maximal ICP, and its relevance is covered in more detail other chapters.

The term *long centric* is often used by clinicians. This, in essence, describes the scenario of being able to close the mandible into the retruded contact position (RCP) (or slightly anterior to it) without altering the vertical dimension of the anterior teeth.[26] The presence and direction of any slides between RCP and ICP should be noted; this aspect is critical to the planning of restorative rehabilitation of the TW patient, as discussed at length in other chapters.

In the sagittal plane the mandible can only exhibit rotational and translational movement; it has been suggested that rotation is limited to about 12 mm of incisor separation before translational movements of the temporal joint commence. The term *terminal hinge axis* is used to describe an imaginary horizontal line that passes through the rotational centres of each the condylar processes. The practical relevance of the terminal hinge axis is discussed further in Chapter 5.

In relation to the dynamic mandibular movements, it is important to assess the relationships during lateral and protrusive movements. The term *anterior (or incisal) guidance* refers to the guidance provided by the contact formed between the palatal surfaces of the anterior maxillary teeth and their antagonists, whilst the term *protrusive guidance* is used to describe the effect stemming from the combined influence of the condylar guidance (developed between the condyle and fossa during anterior mandibular movement), the *distal guiding component*, and the anterior guidance, the *anterior guiding component*. The average protrusive condylar angle is 45° (range of 30–60°). Where the occlusal scheme is considered to be *stable* (*mutually protective*), when the patient displays a protrusive mandibular movement, the anterior guidance coupled with the inclination of the condylar path should collectively aim to separate (or disclude) the posterior teeth from each other, thereby avoiding any harmful occlusal contacts which may otherwise culminate in cuspal fractures, repeated restoration fracture, recurrent decementation of indirect restorations, pathological tooth wear or fremitus. However, in the position of maximum intercuspation only light occlusal contacts should exist between the anterior segments, with occlusal loading primarily taking place between the posterior teeth.

The steepness of the anterior guidance provided by the anterior teeth should also be recorded as being steep, moderate or shallow. The effect of altering the anterior guidance on the posterior dentition must be carefully evaluated where the clinician may be contemplating a macroscopically irreversible alteration in the anterior guidance, such as the prescription of multiple anterior crowns. Ideally, the anterior guidance should be shared between the anterior teeth to optimise stress distribution, but this may not always be possible.[26] Clearly, however, the steeper the anterior guidance, the more likely it is that posterior disclusion will take place.

The lateral movement of the mandible is analogously influenced by the tooth relationships as well as the condyle-fossa arrangement during the undertaking of such movements. Occlusal contacts when undertaking *mandibular lateral excursive movements* should also be assessed; the term *working side* is used to refer to the direction in which the mandible has moved during a lateral excursion, with the alternative being the *non-working* si*de*. Lateral guidance may be provided by the canine teeth *canine guidance* or by multiple teeth, referred to as *group function*. The morphology of the canine tooth makes it a very suitable candidate to provide guidance during lateral excursive movements. The presence of a *canine-guided occlusion/canine protected occlusion* helps to permit posterior tooth disclusion upon lateral excursion, which may otherwise lead to similar disastrous consequences, as discussed above. It is also common to observe a relationship which may initially involve group function, but the presence of canine guidance is noted at the end of the lateral excursive movement.

Determining cuspal guidance is largely dependent on the body position of the patient as for the majority of subjects (96%) dynamic occlusal contacts change when body position is altered.[27] During life it can be expected that canine guidance will change into a group function. However, it has yet not been proven that for TW canine guidance is 'protective' for the other teeth. With reference to the condyle-fossa relationships that take place during the process of making a lateral excursive movement, the principle movement within the TMJs is on the *non-working side* (the side away from which the mandible moves in lateral excursion).[28] During this action, the head of the condyle moves forwards, downwards, and medially. The angle of medial movement is referred to as the *Bennet angle* and has an average value of 7.5°. The movement that takes place at the working side is referred to as the *immediate side shift* or *Bennett movement*. The average level of lateral movement is approximately 1 mm.

A number of alternative occlusal schemes have been described in the literature, such as *balanced occlusion (bilaterally balanced occlusion)* and *unilaterally balanced occlusion*. The former is used to describe a relationship recommended when undertaking complete denture prosthodontics to ensure denture stability during dynamic movements.

The presence of any *occlusal interference* (undesirable contacts that occur between opposing teeth in any mandibular position), which may cause mandibular displacement on either the working side (the side towards which the mandible moves during a lateral excursive movement) or the non-working side (the side away from which the mandible moves in lateral excursion), should also be noted. When undertaking restorative rehabilitation involving a reorganised approach, in the ideal situation lateral guidance should be provided by the canine teeth, with the absence of any occlusal interference on either the working side or non-working side. However, it is important to appreciate that the presence of non-working side contacts (when not associated with the presence of signs or symptoms of pathology) does not constitute the presence of an occlusal interference; such contacts may be seen amongst patients with malocclusions or natural occlusal schemes that do not otherwise conform to the mechanical ideal.

The topic of clinical occlusion in relation to the management of the worn dentition is discussed further in Chapter 5.

3.5.2.5 Evaluation of the Aesthetic Zone

The terms *aesthetic zone* or *smile zone* are often applied in the literature to denote the appearance of the teeth and smile. Indeed, as discussed above, matters relating to aesthetic impairment are the most common cause for a patient to express concerns in relation to a wearing dentition. It is thus paramount to undertake a meticulous assessment of the aesthetic zone during patient examination to help best determine which features may require addressing when developing the treatment plan.[29]

Analysis of the aesthetic zone should aim to evaluate the features described in the following sections.

3.5.2.5.1 *The Dento-labial Relationships*

The term *lip line* or *smile line* is used to describe the relationship that exists between the inferior border of the upper lip and teeth and the gingival soft tissues on smiling (or when asked to make an 'e' sound). Three types of lip line are commonly described:

- *low smile line*: where the motility of the upper lip exposes the anterior teeth by no more than 75%, with no display of gingival tissue (low smile lines can be the most forgiving in cases of restorative imperfections)
- *medium smile line*: where lip movement culminates in the display of between 75% and 100% of the anterior teeth as well as the interdental papillae
- *high smile line*: which exposes the teeth in full in display as well as the gingival tissues beyond the gingival margins, often referred to as a 'gummy smile'.

The *width of the smile* should also be analysed. For optimum aesthetics, the dental hard tissues should fill the corners, avoiding the presence of *negative buccal corridors*.

The *smile arc* should also be evaluated. This describes the relationship that exists between the curvature of the lower lip to the curvature of the incisal edges of the maxillary incisor teeth in a posed smile. Ideally, the curvature of the lower lip should be parallel to that of the incisor edges and the superior border of the lower lip be spatially positioned slightly inferior to the incisal edges. This information can be used to plan the appropriate design of any future restorations, especially when undertaking rehabilitation of a severely worn anterior maxillary dentition.

3.5.2.5.2 The Dental Midlines

Ideally, the dental midline should coincide with the facial midline. The maxillary centre line is best evaluated against the midpoint of the philtrum; a discrepancy of up to 2 mm between the maxillary midline and the facial midline may be considered aesthetically acceptable. The mandibular midline should ideally be coincident with the maxillary midline. However, this feature has been observed to occur physiologically only amongst 25% of the population.

3.5.2.5.3 Tooth Colour and Form

Tooth colour: Teeth should be evaluated for variations in colour:

- hue – basic colour
- chroma – saturation of the basic colour
- value – brightness

Tooth form: The form of the maxillary central incisors (ovoid, square or triangular) has been suggested (without any scientific basis) to reflect the personality, sex, age, and strength index of a particular individual. Tooth form may also alter with age as a result of TW. In the absence of any information relating to the likely morphology of the anterior teeth prior to ascertaining wear, the use of such information may help determine an appropriate tooth form.

3.5.2.5.4 Tooth Size, Proportion, Shape, Symmetry, Position, and Axial Inclination

The maxillary central incisor teeth are generally accepted as the most dominant teeth in the aesthetic zone, with reported average length and width of 10–11 mm and 8–9 mm, respectively,[30] and a height to base ratio of 1.2 : 1. It is also frequently stated that the central incisor length should be approximately one-sixteenth of the facial height. Knowledge of these baseline values may help to plan the restoration of severely worn anterior dentition.

In cross-sectional profile the maxillary central incisor teeth typically present with two or three planes on the labial face. Over-contouring in the labial-gingival portion (frequently seen as a consequence of restorative intervention) may result in not only poor aesthetics, but also the initiation of periodontal disease.

The mathematical concept of the *golden proportion* is used by some practitioners. It suggests an ideal proportion of 1 : 1.618, thus in the context of anterior maxillary dentition this implies that the maxillary central incisor should be 1.6 times wider than the maxillary lateral incisor, which in turn would be 1.6 times wider than the maxillary canine when viewed from a frontal direction.[31] Accordingly, the width of the maxillary canine should be 62% of the width of the lateral incisor, which itself would be 62% of the width of the maxillary central incisor. The golden proportion, however, has been shown to exist in less than 20% of all natural dentitions examined.[32]

Minor levels of asymmetry between the maxillary central incisors are more commonly observed than perfect symmetry. It is also desirable for the morphology of the disto-incisal line angles of the anterior maxillary teeth to have a symmetrical appearance. The presence of peg-shaped lateral incisors or indeed absent teeth may have a profound effect on the symmetrical arrangement of the anterior maxillary region.

When viewed from a frontal direction, the anterior maxillary teeth have a tendency towards a mesial tilt or inclination towards the vertical midline. The angle of inclination increases in moving laterally from the central incisors to the canines. A noticeable lack of symmetry in the axial inclination of the anterior teeth may culminate in a poor aesthetic appearance.

Again, each of the above concepts may be applied when designing a *new aesthetic zone* where the existing features may have been markedly affected by the process of TW.

3.5.2.5.5 Contact Areas, Connectors, and Embrasures

According to the universally accepted concepts in dental aesthetics, *embrasure spaces* should ideally increase in size in progressing distally away from the midline, whilst *contact points* should be positioned in a more apical location when moving distally from the midline in a symmetrical manner.

The *connector* may be defined as 'the area between two adjacent teeth that seem to touch in a frontal view'.[33] Dias et al. have suggested the application of the 50–40–30 rule in defining the aesthetic relationship between the anterior maxillary teeth, whereby the ideal connector area between the central incisors is 50% of the length of their clinical crowns, the length between the central incisor and lateral incisors is 40% of the length of the crown of the central incisor, and 30% of the length of the central incisor tooth between the lateral incisor and canine teeth, respectively.[33] Connectors should ideally be symmetrical across the dental midline.

3.5.2.5.6 Gingival Aesthetics

The gingival levels of the anterior maxillary segment should ideally be symmetrical about the midline, with the horizontal gingival levels of the central incisor and canine teeth being placed slightly more apical (by approximately 1 mm) than that of the lateral incisors. The gingival biotype should also be determined (subclassified as being thick or thin) as this may influence how the gingival tissues respond to surgical procedures or the placement of future dental restorations.

Figure 3.6 provides a resume of the features that should be appraised and recorded as part of the aesthetic zone assessment.

3.5.2.6 Assessment of any Edentulous Areas

Where any edentulous spaces may be present, it is conventional to provide a spatial description of them. A number of classification systems have been proposed to assist with this process. In the UK, the *Kennedy classification system* is frequently used. This takes into account the location of the saddle(s) (as being anterior or posterior), whether they are unbounded (unilaterally or bilaterally), and/or whether any bounded saddles may be present. Where multiple edentulous spaces are present within single arch, each additional space is termed a 'modification'.

Edentulous areas should be assessed for their overall form, often ascribed as being 'rounded', 'flat', 'inverted' or 'knife edged'/'sharp', and the overlying mucosa examined for consistency as to whether it is 'firmly bound' or 'flabby/

displaceable'. The other denture bearing tissues should also be examined and a note made of the presence of any *hard or soft tissue undercuts*.

Any existing removable prostheses should be assessed for retention, stability, support, base form, polished surface contours, occlusal prescription, and aesthetics.

The prosthodontic rehabilitation of any edentulous spaces in a patient presenting with TW may be of greater importance, especially if there is a need to improve the distribution of occlusal loads to improve the longevity of the residual dentition.

Figure 3.7 provides a summary of the aspects that are usually assessed and recorded during this part of the examination.

3.6   Special Tests

Special tests are routinely prescribed in dentistry to help derive a diagnosis. Special tests commonly performed for patients with TW may include the following:

- *Radiographs*: Good-quality, accurate, paralleled periapical radiographs are advocated for any teeth displaying signs of wear and also for any teeth where active restorative intervention may be being considered. It is important to establish the presence of any signs of alveolar bone loss to help establish a periodontal diagnosis. Other features that may also be elicited upon radiography include the root surface morphology, the anatomy of the pulp chambers of affected teeth, the quality of pre-existing endodontic treatment(s), the presence of dental caries, and widening/disturbance of the lamina dura. The presence of retained roots or any signs of periapical pathology (radiolucencies or radio-opacities) should also be assessed.
- *Articulated study casts*: Good-quality study casts will permit an assessment of the occlusion in the absence of soft tissue/muscular interferences. For further details, see Chapter 5.
- *Digital 3D scans*: Three-dimensional images of both jaws include bite registration. This gives much more detail and contrast in comparison to traditional casts.
- *Sensibility tests*: As discussed above, undiagnosed apical pathology may be present in approximately one-tenth of teeth displaying signs of severe wear.[6,7] It is therefore appropriate to establish the periapical and pulp tissue health of affected teeth, especially when contemplating prosthodontic rehabilitation. Indeed, one frequently cited study in the dental literature has reported the risk of irreversible pulp tissue damage following the preparation of a tooth to receive a full coverage crown to be 19%.[33] However, it has since been suggested that a more realistic estimation of the loss of vitality following the preparation and provision of crown restoration is 4–8% in the 10 years following active treatment.[34]

Given the heightened risks for the presence of reversible or irreversible pulpitis at teeth with severe wear coupled with the further copious loss of tooth tissue and the additional stresses that may be re-laid to the pulp tissues by the processes of tooth preparation and crown cementation, respectively, the risks for developing apical periodontitis at such teeth in the view of the authors is likely to be greater (than that for teeth that do not display signs of severe wear).

Sensibility tests together with clinical and radiographic observations are traditionally used in general practice to carry out pulp tissue assessments. Sensibility tests may typically involve the application of ethyl chloride, warmed gutta percha, and/or electric stimuli to the tooth. However, the *'true' vitality status* of a tooth can strictly be only established with the use of more complex measures, such as the use of Doppler flow techniques.

- *Intra-oral photographs* can provide an excellent means of communication, as well as an invaluable form of dental record. Photographs should include (at least) an anterior view, posterior (left/right) views, and occlusal views of both arches.
- *Salivary analysis* can be undertaken for both stimulated and unstimulated secretion rates and respective buffering capacities, especially in cases where discrepancies with saliva secretion may serve as a potential co-factor.

3.7 Summary

Having systematically carried out the above assessment and evaluations, the clinician will be in a position to assemble a 'problem list', perhaps better referred to as a diagnosis or a differential diagnosis. This can be disseminated into recognised logical sequences for treatment planning (as discussed in Chapter 9) to approach care in a systematic manner, with the aim of providing the patient with the most predictable and favourable long-term outcome. The assessments will also help to determine an overall risk assessment, which may be used to tailor future treatment needs.

3.8 Conclusion

Treatment planning for a patient displaying signs of TW can be challenging, especially if restorative rehabilitation is to be undertaken. It is imperative that an appropriate diagnosis/diagnoses is established. The latter (as described above) requires a comprehensive patient assessment, which may sometimes take several attendances to complete.

In Chapter 4 details will be provided concerning using the information gathered to determine a diagnosis, including the manner in which the severity, extent, and location of TW may be described, such as by the use of clinical indices.

Name: Date of assessment:

Patient complaint(s) (aesthetic, functional, symptoms, concerns with TW/ failing restorations); / desires, expectations:

-

History of present complaint: ....

Relevant MH/ Drugs/ Allergies:
-
-

Relevant Social History:

Smoker: Y/N   How many / day?...   How long Yrs.....
Alcohol: Y/N   Units / week?.......
Occupation ....
Psychological stress levels (0–10) ....
Recreational habits of note ....

Diet:

- Sugar intake: Hot drinks   Cakes Biscuits Sweets
                        Others:

- Acid intake: Carbonated drinks   Fresh fruit   Fruit juices
                        Others:

- Methods of food/beverage consumption ....

Past Dental History:

Last dental visit: .... Regular dental attender: Y/N

OH Regime: ETB   Yes.... No.... Tooth brush texture: Dentifrice used:
                        Interspace   Yes.... No....
                        Floss   Yes.... No....
                        Mouthwash/ Fl agents being used ....

Other notes: (history of awareness of clenching/ grinding habit/ splint use)
....

Figure 3.1 Extract from an assessment template used to gather further patient history.

Extra-oral examination:

- Maximum opening   Inter-incisal distance..................mm/ Range of Lateral movement ....mm/

- Joints sounds   Y/N - Click; single/ multiple   Early/ Later   Other sounds/ anomalies

- Muscle/ Joint tendernes   Yes...   No...

- Signs of Hyposalivation: Y/N

- Facial Proportions/ well balanced: Y/N – comments: OVD: mm/   RVD: mm/   FWS: mm/

- Facial Profile: Normal/ Convex/ Concave

- Facial Symmetry: Horizontal: Y/N   Vertical: Y/N

- Facial Shape: Square/ Ovoid/ Tapering/Square Tapering

- Lip mobility: Incisor display on smiling: mm/

Figure 3.2 Recording relevant extra-oral findings.

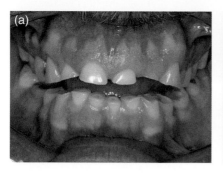 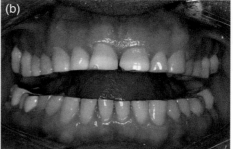

Figure 3.3 (a) Patient with generalised tooth wear with compensatory alveolar growth. (b) Patient with severe generalised tooth wear without compensatory alveolar growth.

Intra-oral examination

- Soft tissues   Linea alba   ....

  Tongue faceting   ....

  Gingival biotype   thick / thin

  Other   ....

- BPE:

  0 No bleeding or pocketing >3.5 mm detected

  1 Bleeding on probing - no pocketing > 3.5 mm

  2 Plaque retentive factors; supra/subgingival calculus/ overhangs present - no pocketing > 3.5 mm

  3 Pockets > 3.5 mm but < 5.5mm in depth; indicating pocket of 4–5 mm

  4 Pockets > 5.5 mm in depth; indicating pocket of 6 mm or more.

  (* - furcation involvement)

- Mobility, Recession and Furcation Involvement:

P																	P
F																	F
R																	R
M																	M
	8	7	6	5	4	3	2	1	1	2	3	4	5	6	7	8	
	8	7	6	5	4	3	2	1	1	2	3	4	5	6	7	8	
M																	M
R																	R
F																	F
P																	P

- Hard Tissues

8 7 6 5 4 3 2 1   1 2 3 4 5 6 7 8

- Significant findings (caries, fracture, wear)

....

....

Figure 3.4 Soft tissue, hard tissue, and periodontal findings relevant to the intra-oral examination.

(*Continued*)

	sextant 1		sextant 2		sextant 3	
	occlusal		incisal		occlusal	
			sextant 2			
			palatinal			
	sextant 6		sextant 5		sextant 4	
	occlusal		incisal		occlusal	

Figure 3.4 (Continued)

<u>Occlusion</u>

Skeletal Pattern: I/ II / III

Incisal Relationship   I / II div /   div 2/ III

OJ = ...mm

OB = ...mm   complete / incomplete

Over eruptions: ....

Tilting: ....

Spacing: ....

Crowding: ....

Drifting: ....

Number of tooth contacts (shimstock holds)   ....

Loss of posterior support .... Y/N

ICP = RCP /   ICP ≠ RCP   Slide: vertical: horizontal:

First point of contact (RCP): ....

Dynamic features/ Guidance (chart teeth)

    Protrusion:

      Lateral excursion: Left: Right:

               Canine guidance   ...   Canine guidance   ...
               Group function   ...   Group function   ...

               NWSI...............   NWSI.............

Figure 3.5 Summary of the features that should be assessed and recorded as part of the occlusal assessment.

- Smile line: High (100% of incisors / all gingiva visible)   ....

                            Medium (75–100% of incisors / papilla visible)   ....

                            Low (<75% of incisors / no gingiva visible)   ....

- Smile arc: Parallelism between the lower lip and anterior maxillary plane .... Y/N
- Negative buccal corridor .... Y/N
- Symmetry
    - Between facial midline and dental maxillary) midline ...... Y/N   Comments: ....
    - Between the maxillary arch and mandibular arch .... Y/N   Comments: ....
    - Between teeth across the maxillary midline .... Y/N   Comments: ....
- Length/ width of central incisor teeth R; length ....mm/ width.......mm/ L; length ....mm/ width ......mm/
- Colour/ shade ....
- Other notes ....

Figure 3.6 Assessment of the aesthetic zone.

Maxilla:

Kennedy Classification:

Edentulous Span:

Alveolar Ridge: Resorption   vertical / horizontal

                            Firm / Flabby / Round / Flat / Sharp / Undercut

Tuberosity:

Palate:

Potential Abutments:

Mandible:

Kennedy Classification:

Edentulous Span:

Alveolar Ridge: Resorption   vertical / horizontal

                            Firm / Flabby/ Round / Flat / Sharp / Undercut

Lingual concavity

Potential Abutments:

Existing Dentures:

Maxilla:

Mandible:

Figure 3.7 Summary of the edentulous space assessment.

References

1 Banerji, S., Mehta, S.B., and Ho, C.K. (2017). *Practical Procedures in Aesthetic Dentistry*. Wiley Blackwell.
2 Kelleher, M., Bomfim, D., and Austin, R. (2012). Biologically based restorative management of tooth wear. *Int. Jour. Dent.* 2012: 1–9.
3 Slater, L., Eder, A., and Wilson, N. (2016). Worning: tooth wear ahead. *Prim. Dent. J.* 5 (3): 38–42.
4 Loomans, B., Opdam, N., Attin, T. et al. (2017). Severe tooth wear: European consensus statement on management guidelines. *J. Adhes. Dent.* 19: 111–119.
5 Ganss, C. (2014). Is tooth wear an oral disease? *Monogr. Oral Sci., Karger* 25: 16–21.
6 Wazani, B., Dodd, M., and Milosevic, A. (2012). The signs and symptoms of tooth wear in a referred group of patients. *Br. Dent. J.* 213: E10.
7 Siasasithamparam, K., Harbrow, D., Vinczer, E., and Young, W. (2003). Endodontic sequelae of dental erosion. *Aust. Dent. J.* 48: 97–101.
8 Slade, G. and Spencer, A. (1994). Development and evaluation of the oral health impact profile. *Community Dent. Health* 11: 3–11.
9 Li, M. and Bernabe, E. (2016). Tooth wear and quality of life among adults in the United Kingdom. *J. Dent.* 55: 48–53.
10 Watson, M. and Burke, F. (2000). Investigation and treatment of patients with teeth affected by tooth substance loss: a review. *Dent. Update* 27: 175–183.
11 Moazzez, R. and Bartlett, D. (2014). Intrinsic causes of erosion. *Monogra. Oral Sci., Karger* 25: 180–196.
12 Lavigne, G., Khoury, S., Abe, S. et al. (2008). Review article: Bruxism physiology and pathology: an overview for clinicians. *J. Oral. Rehabil.* 35 (7): 476–494.
13 Chiang, H., Gau, S., Ni, H. et al. (2010). Association between symptoms and subtypes of attention-deficit hyperactivity disorder and sleep problems/disorders. *J. Sleep Res.* 19 (4): 535–545.
14 Shellis, R. and Addy, M. (2014). The interactions between attrition, abrasion and erosion in tooth wear. *Monogr. Oral Sci., Karger* 25: 32–45.
15 Gray, R. and Al-Ani, Z. (2010). Risk management in clinical practice. Part 8. Temporomandibular disorders. *Br. Dent. J.* 209: 433–449.
16 Scully, C. and Felix, D. (2005). 3: Oral medicine — update for the dental practitioner: dry mouth and disorders of salivation. *Br. Dent. J.* 199: 423–427.
17 Fradeani, M. (2004). Facial analysis. In: *Esthetic Rehabilitation in Fixed Prosthodontics. Volume 1, Esthetic Analysis*, 35–62. Quintessence Books.
18 Abudo, J. and Lyons, K. (2012). Clinical considerations for increasing occlusal vertical dimension: a review. *Aust. Dent. J.* 57: 2–10.
19 Rivera-Morales, W. and Mohl, N. (1993). Restoration of the vertical dimension of the occlusion in the severely worn dentition. *Dent. Clin. N. Am.* 36: 651–663.
20 Ahmad, I. (2005). Anterior dental aesthetics: dentofacial perspective. *Br. Dent. J.* 199: 81–88.
21 Vig, R. and Brundo, G. (1978). The kinetics of anterior tooth display. *J. Prosthet. Dent.* 39: 502–504.
22 The Challacomb Scale (2011). www.challacombescale.co.uk/Challacombe-Scale-ENG.pdf.

23 Hadden, A. (2016). *Clinical Examination & Record Keeping, Good Practice Guidelines*, 3e. FGDP.

24 Baker, P. and Needleman, I. (2010). Risk management in clinical practice. Part 10. Periodontology. *Br. Dent. J.* 209: 557–565.

25 Davies, S., Gray, R., Linden, G., and James, J. (2001). Occlusal considerations in periodontics. *Br. Dent. J.* 191: 597–604.

26 Milosevic, A. (2003). Occlusion: 1. Terms, mandibular movement and the factors of occlusion. *Dent. Update* 30: 359–361.

27 van't Spijker, A., Creugers, N.H., Bronkhorst, E.M., and Kreulen, C.M. (2011). Body position and occlusal contacts in lateral excursions: a pilot study. *Int. J. Prosthodont.* 24 (2): 133–136.

28 Davies, S. and Gray, R. (2001). What is occlusion? *Br. Dent. J.* 191: 235–245.

29 Mehta, S.B., Aulakh, R., and Banerji, S. (2015). Patient assessment: preparing for a predictable aesthetic outcome. *Dent. Update* 42: 78–86.

30 Summit, J., Robbins, J., Hilton, T., and Schwartz, R. (2006). *Fundamentals of Operative Dentistry, a Contemporary Approach*, 3e, 68–80. Quintessence Books.

31 Levin, E. (1978). Dental esthetics and the golden proportion. *J. Prosthet. Dent.* 40: 244–252.

32 Preston, J. (1993). The golden proportion revisited. *J. Esthet. Dent.* 5: 247–251.

33 Dias, N. and Tsingene, F. (2011). SAEF – Smile's aesthetic evaluation form: a useful tool to improve communication between clinicians and patients during multidisciplinary treatment. *Eur. J. Esthet. Dent.* 6: 160–175.

34 Saunders, W. and Saunders, E. (1998). Prevalence of periradicular periodontitis associated with crowned teeth in the adult Scottish subpopulation. *Br. Dent. J.* 185: 137–140.

Further Reading

Horner, K. and Eaton, K. (2013). *Selection criteria for Dental Radiography*, 3e. FGDP.

Mehta, S.B., Banerji, S., Millar, B.J., and Saures-Fieto, J.M. (2012). Current concepts in tooth wear managements. Part 1: assessment, treatment planning and strategies for the prevention and passive monitoring of tooth wear. *Br. Dent. J.* 212 (1): 17–27.

Whitworth, J., Walls, G., and Wassell, R. (2002). Crowns and extra-coronal restorations; endodontic complications: the pulp, the root-treated tooth and the crown. *Br. Dent. J.* 192: 315–327.

4

The Diagnosis of Tooth Wear, Including the Use of Common Clinical Indices

4.1   Introduction

Given the likely progressive growth in the rates of prevalence of tooth wear (TW), coupled with the irreversible loss of tooth tissue that occurs as part of the associated pathological mechanisms (which in some cases may commit the patient to having to be provided with complex and costly dental care),[1] it is important for the dental practitioner to ascertain the presence of TW when carrying out the dental examination of their patients. Accordingly, it is important that a diagnosis of TW is made and appropriate measures taken in an attempt to halt any further disease progression.

Having recognised or qualified the problem of TW in the oral cavity, there is the subsequent need to quantify the pattern of wear present.[1] This involves undertaking a *grading of the severity* of the condition.

The processes of qualifying and quantifying the TW present will enable the clinician to establish a clear, comprehensive, and a reasonably accurate baseline diagnosis which in turn may be used to enable:

- effective communication with the patient
- more meaningful discussions with other dental colleagues (including the need to provide a referral to the secondary or tertiary care sector)
- monitoring of the disease progression (Figure 4.1)
- evaluation of the efficacy of any preventative therapy that may have been prescribed and implemented
- determination of the point in time where restorative intervention may be suitable
- planning of the provision of treatment using established protocols.

The quantification of TW may be carried out using *in vivo* and/or *in vitro* techniques.[1-3] In relation to the use of *in vitro* protocols, there are a number of techniques that can be used. Some of the more sophisticated techniques, which are often not clinically applicable in general dental practice, include:[2]

- scanning electron microscopy and energy-dispersive X-ray spectroscopy
- measuring light microscopy
- surface 3D focus variation scanning microscopy
- attenuated total reflectance infrared spectroscopy

Practical Procedures in the Management of Tooth Wear, First Edition. Subir Banerji, Shamir Mehta, Niek Opdam and Bas Loomans.
© 2020 John Wiley & Sons Ltd. Published 2020 by John Wiley & Sons Ltd.
Companion website: www.wiley.com/go/banerji/toothwear

- optical specular and diffuse reflection analysis
- white light interferometry
- optical coherence tomography
- surface hardness measurements
- surface profilometry
- chemical analysis of the minerals dissolved in the erosive agent
- microradiography and atomic force microscopy
- ultrasound measurements of enamel thickness
- nano indentation
- confocal laser scanning microscopy
- iodide permeability tests
- element analysis of solid samples.

Whilst the use of these techniques would not generally be possible in the primary care setting, other tools are more readily available to the general dental practitioner and may be easily used for the diagnosis of TW. They include the following:

- *High-quality clinical photographs* of standardised views taken at suitable periodical intervals can be used to monitor gross morphological changes, noting factors such as the increase in the translucency and alterations in the shade of a tooth. which may be a sign of thinning enamel.[4]

    Photos should be taken of the occlusal aspect of the maxillary arch (showing the occlusal, incisal, and palatal surfaces of all of the teeth present), the occlusal view of the lower arch (capturing all of the occlusal and incisal surfaces), and frontal and lateral views (of both sides). For the frontal and lateral views, ideally teeth should be parted and the buccal/labial sections of both arches be clearly evident. An index such as the Tooth Wear Evaluation System (TWES)[1,5] can be used in conjunction with high-quality photographs to carry out the grading of wear, especially on occlusal/incisal surfaces.[6]

    Good digital clinical photographs are indispensable in treatment planning, however only using photographs to monitor wear over time is difficult as small differences are very difficult to detect by the naked eye.

- *High-quality dental casts* poured in vacuum-mixed die stone based on accurate impressions taken using appropriate trays and materials,[7] which with the aid of a baseline index prepared from the initial set of casts (using a suitable, dimensionally stable material) can be used to enable comparisons in minor changes in tooth morphology over longer periods of time to be made, or the use of a clinical index such as the Basic Erosive Wear Examination (BEWE), Tooth Wear Index (TWI), or TWES (as discussed below) to monitor changes extra-orally (Figure 4.2).[6]

- *Contemporary digital systems* involving intraoral scanning devices to make digital impressions (which are often used in general dental practice) may be a helpful tool for the purpose of quantification, whereby the use of a 3D scanner may offer the capacity to detect subtle volumetric loss in a sensitive manner (using 3D models and/or casts), and thus prove particularly helpful in monitoring progression, especially for cases with very mild (early stage) erosive wear (Figures 4.3 and 4.4).[3,4] Digital models can also be printed in plastic (stereolithography apparatus models).

- *Scratch tests* involving the use of a small quantity of flowable resin composite or a low-viscosity addition cured silicone material (supported by a wooden tongue spatula) to take an impression of a line scored across an affected tooth using a number 12 scalpel blade may also be performed. This process is repeated 1–4 weeks thereafter, with the aim of viewing the changes using suitable magnification to effectively to ascertain the rate of disappearance of the groove in the impression medium.[8] In the author's opinion this test will require specific patient consent and acceptance of this method of monitoring may be low.

It is important to clinically quantify the level of wear present once its presence has been established. This is, however, by no means a straightforward task primarily due to a lack of consensus (often with terminology and the available indices), as well as the sensitivity of the generally available means to determine the extent and severity of TW present.

This is perhaps made more apparent by taking the example of quantifying the effects of chronic periodontal disease as a comparison, where there appears to be a consensus on the means by which the level of disease experience can be diagnosed and recorded. Such means include the evaluation of the overall standard of oral hygiene, the undertaking of probing depth assessments, determining the levels of recession, bleeding on probing, the presence and severity of any tooth mobility, furcation involvement etc. However, in the case of TW, there is a far lower level of consensus, with some clinicians preferring a more descriptive means of reporting and recording, whilst others may prefer the use of an approved *clinical index*, or indeed a combination approach.

This chapter explores the means by which the *location and severity* of the presenting pattern of wear can be further described and suitably documented, as well as briefly considering the limitations that the current, more readily accessible methods of diagnosing and recording the levels of TW pose.

4.2   The Use of Descriptive Means to Qualify and Quantify Tooth Wear

According to Wetselaar and Lobbezoo,[1] *qualification* of TW is an important step in the diagnostic process, whereby an effort should be made to determine the subtype of wear (*attrition, erosion or abrasion*) based on the clinical appearance of the lesions seen. For further details concerning the clinical appearance of the lesions associated with these processes, refer to Chapter 3. However, as also eluded to in Chapter 3, TW more often than not involves multifactorial processes, rendering it (at times) very challenging to establish the likely causes, especially when the process of wear may be considered to be severe. For this reason, a classification system has been described to embrace the most likely origin of wear for a given sextant in the following manner:[1]

- mechanical/intrinsic (attrition)
- mechanical/extrinsic (abrasion)
- chemical/intrinsic (erosion)
- chemical/extrinsic (erosion).

Ideally, an effort should also be made to determine if the pattern of wear observed is likely to suggest a condition is *active* or *quiescent*. Meyers has described a number of clinical indicators that may be associated with active lesions and may prove to be a helpful guide in making this assessment.[9] These include the following:

- decreased surface lustre on enamel and dentine, which may serve as an indicator for acid dissolution of the tooth surface, akin to what may be seen following the application of an acid etchant
- lack of reflectivity of the tooth surface upon gentle air drying
- dentine hypersensitivity due to dissolution of the smear layer and the opening of dentinal tubules, thereby allowing tubular fluid flow and sensitivity to the applied stimulus (especially in response to acidic food and beverages)
- the absence of calculus, which may be a sign of the presence of unsaturated saliva with a lack of ability to mineralise; the formation of calculus will not occur where there is a balance in favour of demineralisation in the oral cavity.

As a means for providing a summary, and a tool that may prove helpful in clinical practice, the criteria for the *qualification of wear* based on the presenting clinical signs and symptoms are listed in Table 4.1.[1] The content of this table is based on work by Gandara and Truelove,[10] and Ganss and Lussi,[11] and in fact is used as part of the TWES, a modular protocol proposed by Wetselaar et al. to help with the diagnosis of any TW that may be present.[1,5] The TWES is discussed further below.

As part of the process of quantifying the level of TW present, there is a need to determine and suitably document its location and severity.

In relation to the *location* of the pattern of observed wear, when using descriptive processes it is not uncommon to simply list affected teeth using a traditional dental charting system and/or to describe the location as being *localised* or *generalised*.

In the case of a patient presenting with localised TW (comprising one or two sextants),[1] the traditional approach has been to subclassify the pattern by the arch (maxillary or mandibular), as well as by the overall location within the arch (anterior or posterior) or alternatively use a *sextant approach* adopted as per the TWES (Figure 4.5).[1] The latter subdivides the oral cavity into sextants that are subsequently ascribed numbers, hence:

- sextant 1 – upper right posterior (premolars and molars)
- sextant 2 – upper anterior (incisors and canine teeth)
- sextant 3 – upper left posterior
- sextant 4 – lower left posterior
- sextant 5 – lower anterior
- sextant 6 – lower right posterior.

Table 4.1 A summary of the findings that can be used to qualify TW as part of the TWES.[1]

Clinical signs of extrinsic and intrinsic chemical wear
1. Occlusal cupping, incisal grooving, cratering, rounding of cusps and grooves
2. Wear on non-occluding surfaces
3. Raised restorations
4. Broad concavities within the smooth surface enamel, convex areas flatten, or concavities become present, width exceed depth
5. Increased incisal translucency
6. Clean, non-tarnished appearance of amalgams
7. Preservation of enamel cuff in gingival crevice
8. No plaque, discolouration or tartar
9. Hypersensitivity
10. Smooth silky-shining, silky glazed appearance, sometimes dull surface

Clinical signs of intrinsic mechanical wear
1. Shiny facets, flat and glossy
2. Enamel and dentine wear at the same rate
3. Matching wear on occluding surfaces, corresponding features at the antagonistic teeth
4. Possible fracture of restorations
5. Impressions in cheek, tongue and/or lip

Clinical signs of extrinsic mechanical wear
1. Usually located at cervical areas of teeth
2. Lesions more wide than deep
3. Premolars and cuspids are commonly affected

For cases of *generalised tooth wear* (involving three to six sextants),[1] it is also good practice to determine and categorise the amount of dento-alveolar compensation that may have taken place. The loss of tooth structure may or may not result in an increase in the freeway space (FWS). Following an evaluation of the existing occlusal vertical dimension (OVD), as described in Chapter 3, patients presenting with generalised wear may be assigned to three categories according to Turner and Misserilian:[12]

- *Category 1*: Excessive wear with loss of vertical dimension of occlusion.
- *Category 2*: Excessive wear without loss of vertical dimension of occlusion, but with space available.
- *Category 3*: Excessive wear without loss of vertical dimension, but with limited space.

A slower rate of wear with secondary supra-eruption of the dento-alveolar processes is thought to be responsible for contributing to the occurrence of wear in patients in categories 2 and 3. The above classification has a paramount bearing on the restorative strategy adopted, as discussed in detail in Chapter 14.

Traditionally, when attempting to describe the severity of the observed pattern of wear, the use of the terms *physiological wear* and *pathological wear* have commonly been employed. These terms are defined and discussed in Chapter 1. In summary, it is appropriate to note the definition of *pathological tooth wear* as per the European Consensus Statement on the Management Guidelines for Severe Tooth Wear to allay any ambiguity with the use of historical interpretations of these terms, and thereby permit consistency between clinicians. Accordingly, pathological TW has been defined as 'tooth wear which is atypical for the age of the patient, causing pain or discomfort, functional problems, or deterioration of aesthetic appearance, which, if it progresses, may give rise to undesirable complications of increasing complexity'.[13]

In an analogous manner, there has been inconsistency in the means by which the level of severity of the TW may be described. For instance, an approach adopted by Wazani et al.[14] when attempting to determine the prevalence of the signs and symptoms of patients referred to a UK-based dental hospital and described the extent of the presenting TW as being *mild* (for teeth with wear with enamel loss only; Figure 4.6), *moderate* (for teeth displaying the concomitant exposure of dentine) or *severe* (for teeth showing secondary dentine/pulpal exposure; Figure 4.7). Interestingly, the authors of this study also made note of other variables in conjunction with a diagnosis of TW, such as the number of posterior tooth contacts, the number of teeth present, the number of posterior teeth missing, and the Angle classification of the malocclusion. In contrast, however, the BEWE,[15] as discussed at depth below, assigns a sextant score of 3 (on a scale of 0–3, with progressive severity associated with a higher score) on the basis of 'hard tissue loss 50% of the surface loss', whilst others have described the varying levels of severity in the following manner:[1]

- *Mild*: wear within the enamel; occlusal/ incisal and/or non-occlusal/ non-incisal
- *Moderate*: wear with dentine exposure; occlusal/ incisal and/or non-occlusal/ non-incisal
- *Severe*: wear with dentine exposure or loss of clinical crown height less than two-thirds; occlusal/ incisal and/or non-occlusal/non-incisal
- *Extreme*: wear with dentine exposure and loss of clinical crown height at or greater than two-thirds of the crown height; occlusal/incisal regardless of non-occlusal/non-incisal wear.

Therefore, as a means of providing consistency, Loomans et al. have provided a definition of *severe wear* as part of their Consensus Statement as 'tooth wear with substantial loss of tooth structure, with dentine exposure and significant loss (equal to or more than one-third) of the clinical crown'.[13] The importance of consistency is paramount when attempting to make an accurate diagnosis.

The reduction in the height of the clinical crown of an anterior tooth may also be used to ascertain the level of anterior tooth tissue loss. This can be done by taking the distance from the incisal edge to the cemento-enamel junction using a periodontal probe and making a comparison with average values or prior recordings (to ascertain progression or quiescence), as suggested by the TWES.[1]

4.3   The Use of Clinical Indices for the Diagnosis of TW

Many dental practitioners are familiar with the use of clinical indices for the purposes of screening for oral disease, applying various grading systems to evaluate the severity of the presenting condition and using the outcomes to help plan future care needs (applying established guidance). A good example is the Basic Periodontal Examination (BPE), which is widely (and routinely) used in the UK.[16] The use of an analogous index for the purpose of diagnosing TW should ideally offer the clinician the following:

- *A simple, efficient and time effective method to screen for the presence of TW.*
- A clear delineation of the categories to allow the severity to be recorded with minimal intra- and inter-examiner variability, with a level of sensitivity that allows for the monitoring of subtle changes over a period of time.
- A means for determining progression and/or quiescence.
- A protocol based on the use of the index that permits the planning of future care needs.
- Ease of keeping appropriate documentation.

A number of indices have been proposed to grade the severity of TW seen by recording the surface characteristics of teeth with a numerical score and these have gained international approval. However, currently there is no universally accepted index for the recording of TW in general dental practice, neither is there a readily available means to determine whether the presenting activity of the wear process is indeed progressive or quiescent.

Historically, it has generally been considered that the most popular index is the *TWI*, proposed by Smith and Knight.[17] The TWI essentially comprises a five-point scale in which the various tooth surfaces are visually evaluated (cervical, buccal/labial, incisal/occlusal, lingual/palatal). A summary of grades and criteria associated with the use of this index are listed in Table 4.2. Whilst the TWI can

Table 4.2   Tooth wear index by Smith and Knight.[17]

Grade	Criteria
0	No loss of enamel surface characteristics
1	Loss of enamel surface characteristics
2	Buccal, lingual, and occlusal loss of enamel, exposing dentine for less than one-third of the surface Incisal loss of enamel Minimal dentine exposure
3	Buccal, lingual, and occlusal loss of enamel, exposing dentine for more than one-third of the surface Incisal loss of enamel Substantial loss of dentine
4	Buccal, lingual, and occlusal complete loss of enamel, pulp exposure or exposure of secondary dentine Incisal pulp exposure or exposure of secondary dentine

be used to compare wear rates between individuals and also monitor the progression of wear for the patient concerned, it should be noted that this index was initially designed for epidemiological studies and not for the clinical treatment of individual patients.[18]

Indeed, there are a number of other documented drawbacks associated with the routine use of this index, including:[18]

- inter-examiner variability in identifying exposed dentine
- the time taken to administer the index and make recordings
- the exclusion of heavily restored surfaces from the TWI score, rendering it difficult to attain a clear appreciation of the actual level of clinical TW present
- the TWI does not relate the aetiology to the outcome of wear seen on the teeth.

In 2008, Bartlett et al.[15] proposed the *BEWE*, an index aimed at recording the severity of *erosive tooth wear* for patients seen in the primary care setting which would be simple to use, easy to record, create an opportunity to appraise and document that the presence of any TW had been examined/screened for, and, ideally, give future treatment needs due consideration. As an over-arching aim, it was hoped that the undertaking of a BEWE (and documenting the outcomes) would help practitioners to mitigate against claims of supervised neglect (especially in the light of increasing prevalence rates) by demonstrating that an assessment and diagnosis of TW had taken place and been appropriately documented.

The BEWE index is in fact based on the BPE. The latter is a partial scoring system based on a four-point scale widely used in many countries, and as such, given the conceptual parity, it would reasonable to assume that the implementation of the BEWE index in routine clinical practice would pose minimal adaptation for the general practitioner. Indeed, as with the BPE, the BEWE score is recorded on a sextant basis and the value for the worst affected surface for each sextant is recorded.

The protocol/clinical sequence for the use of BEWE as described by Bartlett is as follows:[19]

1) Diagnose the presence of tooth wear, eliminating teeth with trauma and developmental defects from the score.
2) Examine all teeth and all surfaces of teeth in the mouth for tooth wear.
3) Identify in each quadrant the most severely affected tooth with wear.
4) Conduct the BEWE.

The BEWE records the severity of wear on a scale from 0 to 3 for each sextant:

- 0 – No erosive wear
- 1 – Initial loss of surface texture
- 2* – Distinct defect; hard tissue loss less than 50% of the surface area
- 3* – Hard tissue loss equal to or greater than 50% of the surface area.

(*Dentine often involved but may be difficult to detect, especially in the cervical areas.)

On completion of the BEWE, an aggregate *risk assessment score* is reached for all sextants. This score can be used as a means to communicate the patient's level of risk of TW as a guide to the clinical management of the patient concerned.[8,19] The risk score gradings and clinical management guides are summarised in Table 4.3.

There are of course a number of limitations that become apparent with the use of this index; notably, it does not by definition consider the multifactorial aetiology

Table 4.3 BEWE risk score grading and clinical management guide.[8]

Risk level	Cumulative score of all sextants	Management guide
None	Less than or equal to 2	Routine maintenance and observation Review at two yearly intervals
Low	Between 3 and 8	As above plus oral hygiene, dietary assessment, advice Review at two yearly intervals
Medium	Between 9 and 13	As above plus identify main aetiological factors and eliminate Avoid restorations, apply fluorides, casein-derived pastes, surface sealants Monitor at 6–12-month intervals (casts, photos, scratch test)
High	14 and over	As above plus minimal restorations

of TW[1] or enable the measurement of progression, when the changes may be quite subtle.[1] Furthermore, unlike the BPE, which involves the use of a periodontal probe to carry out the screening process, the *in vivo* application of the BEWE is generally based on visual clinical appraisal. Therefore, at times it can be very challenging to clearly distinguish between cases which may not readily fit into scores 2 or 3, with ambiguity over what may be more than or less than 50% surface area loss.

Pragmatic examples of these challenges have been described by Bartlett, such as in the case of TW affecting the entire incisal edge without loss of tooth height.[20] This may cast some doubt over the reliability of this index and perhaps emphasise the importance for examiner calibration to enable its effective application in clinical practice. Indeed, the conclusions of a cross-sectional study carried out by Dixon et al. aimed at appraising the sensitivity, specificity, and reliability of the BEWE stated the index to be effective for the purposes of screening for severe TW, but given their reported moderate levels of examiner reliability, the 'scores should be interpreted with some caution'.[18] It has been shown, however, that the use of the BEWE (as well as the TWES) index can provide a consistent and reliable manner of assessing and monitoring wear with the use of photographs as well as 3D models.[3,6]

It should also be noted that the presence of a relatively higher overall BEWE risk assessment score as a result of localised wear in one sextant may give a distorted representation of the actual pattern of wear present, or a relatively lower score may mask a higher single quadrant score, culminating in the provision of a less than ideal form of management (should the treatment guidelines be strictly adhered to).

For a high-risk factor score of 14 the BEWE prescribes preventive advice, counselling, and monitoring, but it also mentions 'in combination with minimal restorations'. In our opinion additional information is needed to determine whether a restorative intervention is required and this must not be based on an index-score alone.

The BEWE guidance does not indicate clinical management due to the lack of information or help when selecting the most appropriate means of restoring a severely worn dentition. This may be a reflection of the lack of consensus with restorative protocols (although guidance has since been published by Loomans et al. for the appropriate management of such cases).[13]

In an effort to help overcome confusion with how to optimally restore a worn dentition in accordance with the severity of the observed pattern of wear, Vailati and Belser have introduced the *anterior clinical erosive classification (ACE)* based on their clinical observation of the upper anterior teeth.[21]

This classification system has been proposed to not only assess the severity of hard tissue loss but also to provide a guide to the treating clinician on how to appropriately restore the affected teeth. The classification, shown in Table 4.4, establishes six levels of wear according to the level of dentin exposure in the palatal contact areas, the preservation of the incisal edges, the length of the remaining clinical crown, the preservation of enamel on the labial surfaces, and the vitality of the pulp. The *sandwich approach* listed in Table 4.4 refers to the application of a resin-based material to treat the palatal surface wear, followed by the application of a labial/facial ceramic veneer. It should be carefully noted that the guidance is not evidence-based and further work is required to substantiate the efficacy of the suggested protocols and their respective treatment outcomes.

This classification also tries to give restorative advice only based on the amount of lost tooth material. In our opinion such an index may lead to overtreatment as the treatment decision has not been made based on, for example, progression of wear, age of the patient, and, most importantly, if there are functional or esthetical demands from the patient.

Table 4.4 The ACE classification.[21]

Class	Palatal enamel	Palatal dentine	Incisal edge length	Facial enamel	Pulp vitality	Suggested therapy
Class I	Reduced	Not exposed	Preserved	Preserved	Preserved	No restorative treatment, prevention only
Class II	Lost in contact areas	Minimally exposed	Preserved	Preserved	Preserved	Palatal composites
Class III	Lost	Distinctly exposed	Lost ≤2 mm	Preserved	Preserved	Palatal onlays
Class IV	Lost	Extensively exposed	Lost greater than 2 mm	Preserved	Preserved	Sandwich approach
Class V	Lost	Extensively exposed	Lost greater than 2 mm	Distinctly reduced/ lost	Preserved	Sandwich approach (experimental)
Class VI	Lost	Extensively exposed	Lost greater than 2 mm	Lost	Lost	Sandwich approach (highly experimental)

In 2011, Wetsellar et al. proposed the *TWES*, which comprises a *modular based protocol* with the objectives of not only overcoming some of the limitations of the indices described above, but also providing a modular system of appraisal that allows flexibility to enable effective use in both the primary care and referral sector settings.[5] Whilst it is beyond the scope of this textbook to fully describe the TWES modules, it is worth taking note of the screening module used as part of the protocol encompassing the use of a screening tool. As part of this tool, the oral cavity is divided into sextants (as described above) that are *screened twice*, with the first screening being that of the occlusal/incisal surfaces, which are graded using the *five-point ordinal occlusal/incisal grading scale*:

0 No wear
1 Wear confined to enamel
2 Wear with exposed dentine but less than one-third crown height loss
3 Wear greater than one-third but less than two-thirds of crown height loss
4 Wear greater than two-thirds crown height loss.

This is followed by a second sextant grading of the palatal surfaces (based on the premise of their enhanced role in articulation), but now a *three-point ordinal non-occlusal/non-incisal grading scale* is used:

0 No wear
1 Wear confined to enamel
2 Wear with exposed dentine.

Unlike in the BEWE individual sextant scores are not summated.

In summary, a number of indices have been proposed for quantifying the levels of TW present. The most popular ones (TWI, BEWE, and the five-point and three-point ordinal scales) are discussed above. However, there are numerous others that have also been proposed but are perhaps less well known. There is a clear need for an index that will be universally recognised, with fewer limitations (especially in relation to the validity of the diagnostic criteria and grading, notably the relevance and diagnosis of the exposed dentine),[22] that may concomitantly be used with good effect to help plan future treatment needs.

A clinical index may be helpful for the qualification and quantification of TW by expressing the wear as a number, but the relevance of using an index in relation to restorative treatment advice is limited and may even lead to overtreatment.

4.4 Conclusion

There are a number of ways in which a dental practitioner may qualify and quantify the presence of TW. Although there are no universally accepted protocols or indeed a universally accepted index by consensus, it is important that an effort is made to suitably diagnose the presence and extent of any wear affecting a patient, to inform the patient accordingly, and to plan/provide care as deemed necessary to fulfil their healthcare needs. It is likely that the increasing tendency towards the use of intra-oral scanners may in the future provide an effective chairside tool for the diagnosis of TW, as well as the monitoring of its progression.[22]

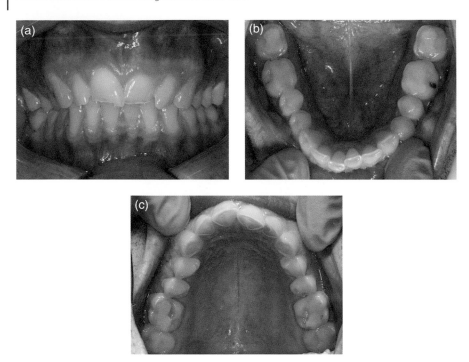

Figure 4.1 Photographs for monitoring TW: (a) labial view with teeth in occlusion, (b) lower occlusal view, and (c) upper occlusal view.

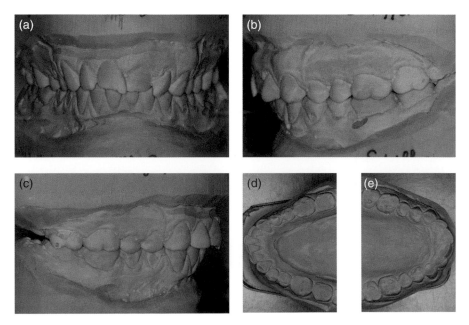

Figure 4.2 Stone casts of the patient shown in Figure 4.1: (a) anterior view with casts in occlusion, (b) left lateral view with casts in occlusion, (c) right lateral view with casts in occlusion, (d) occlusal view of lower cast, and (e) occlusal view of upper cast.

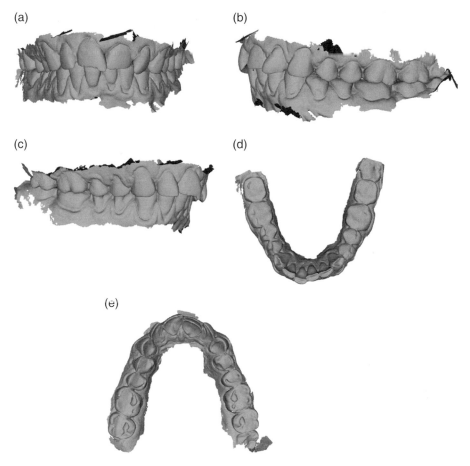

Figure 4.3 Digital scans of the patient shown in Figures 4.1 and 4.2. (a) anterior view with teeth in occlusion, (b) left lateral view with teeth in occlusion, (c) right lateral view with teeth in occlusion, (d) occlusal view of lower teeth, and (e) occlusal view of upper teeth.

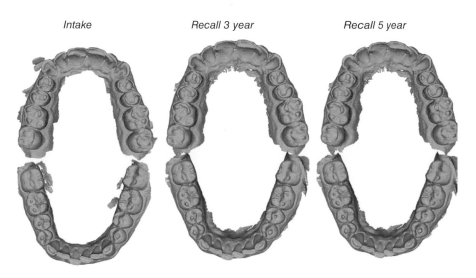

Intake   *Recall 3 year*   *Recall 5 year*

Figure 4.4 TW monitored with sequential digital scans. Male, 44 years old. After 5 years, progression of TW led to functional problems and restorative treatment was started.

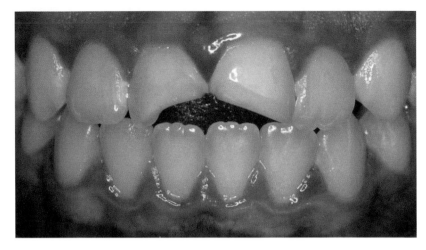

Figure 4.5 Localised TW on the upper central incisors. This patient's TW aetiology is extrinsic chemical in nature. The patient had a habit of using her tongue as a straw to drink acidic soft drinks.

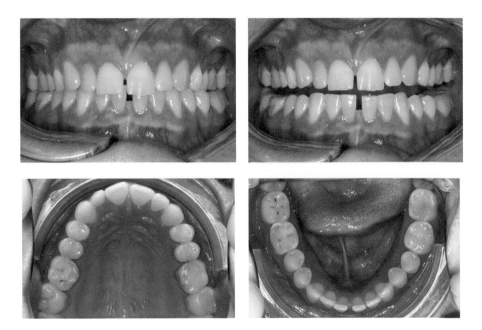

Figure 4.6 Generalised mild TW.

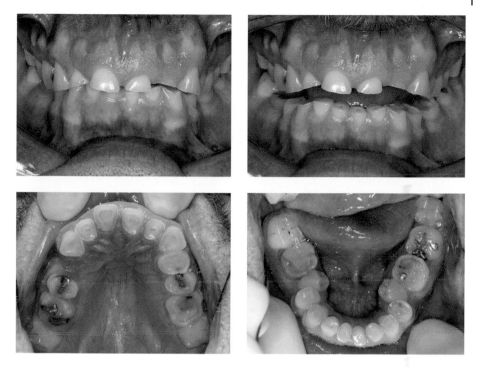

Figure 4.7 Generalised severe TW.

References

1 Wetselaar, P. and Lobbezoo, F. (2016). The tooth wear evaluation system: a modular clinical guideline for the diagnosis and management planning of worn dentitions. *J. Oral Rehabil.* 43: 69–80.
2 Attin, T. and Wegehaupt, F. (2014). Methods for the assessment of dental erosion. *Monogr. Oral Sci., Karger* 25: 123–142.
3 Alaraudanjoki, V., Saarela, H., Pesonen, R. et al. (2017). Is a basic erosive wear examination (BEWE) reliable for recording erosive tooth wear on 3D models? *J. Dent.* 59: 26–32.
4 Ahmed, K., Whitters, J., Ju, X. et al. (2016). A proposed methodology to assess the accuracy of 3D scanners and casts to monitor tooth wear progression in patients. *Int. J. Prosthodont.* 29: 514–521.
5 Wetselaar, P., van der Zaag, J., and Lobbezoo, F. (2011). Tooth wear, a proposal for an evaluation system. *Ned. Tijdschr. Tandheelkd.* 118: 324–328.
6 Wetselaar, P., Wetselaar-Glas, M., Koutris, M. et al. (2016). Assessment of the amount of tooth wear on dental casts and intra-oral photographs. *J. Oral Rehabil.* 43: 615–620.
7 Johansson, A., Johansson, A., Omar, R., and Carlsson, G. (2008). Rehabilitation of the worn dentition. *J. Oral Rehabil.* 35: 548–566.
8 Kaidonis, J. (2012). Oral diagnosis and treatment planning: Part 4. Non-carious tooth surface loss and assessment of risk. *Br. Dent. J.* 213: 155–161.

9 Meyers, I. (2013). Minimum intervention dentistry and the management of tooth wear in general practice. *Aust. Dent. J.* 58 (1): 60–65.

10 Gandara, B. and Truelove, E. (1999). Diagnosis and management of dental erosion. *J. Contemp. Dent. Pract.* 1: 16–23.

11 Ganss, C. and Lussi, A. (2014). Diagnosis of erosive tooth wear. *Monogr. Oral Sci.* 25: 22–31.

12 Rivera-Morales, W. and Mohl, N. (1993). Restoration of the vertical dimension of the occlusion in the severely worn dentition. *Dent. Clin. N. Am.* 36: 651–663.

13 Loomans, B., Opdam, N., Attin, T. et al. (2017). Severe tooth wear: European consensus statement on management guidelines. *J. Adhes. Dent.* 19: 111–119.

14 Wazani, B., Dodd, M., and Milosevic, A. (2012). The signs and symptoms of tooth wear in a referred group of patients. *Br. Dent. J.* 213: E10.

15 Bartlett, D., Ganss, C., and Lussi, A. (2008). Basic erosive wear examination (BEWE): a new scoring system for scientific and clinical needs. *Clin. Oral Investig.* 12 (S1): S65–S68.

16 Basic Periodontal Examination (2016). The British Society of Periodontology. www.bsperio.org.uk.

17 Smith, B. and Knight, J. (1984). An index for measuring the wear of teeth. *Br. Dent. J.* 156: 435–438.

18 Dixon, B., Sharif, M., Ahmed, F. et al. (2012). Evaluation of the basic erosive wear examination (BEWE) for use in general dental practice. *Br. Dent. J.* 213: E4.

19 Bartlett, D. (2010). A proposed system for screening tooth wear. *Br. Dent. J.* 208 (S): 207–209.

20 Bartlett, D. (2016). A personal perspective and update on erosive tooh wear – 10 years on: Part 1 – Diagnosis and prevention. *Br. Dent. J.*: 115–119.

21 Vailati, F. and Belser, U. (2010). Classification and treatment of the anterior maxillary dentition affected by dental erosion: the ACE classification. *Int. J. Periodontics Restorative Dent.* 30: 559–571.

22 Ganss, C. (2014). Is tooth Wear an Oral disease? *Monogr. Oral Sci., Karger* 25: 16–21.

5

Clinical Occlusion in Relation to Tooth Wear

5.1   Introduction

An overview of certain key features in relation to clinical occlusion was provided in Chapter 3, including:

- the importance of undertaking an occlusal assessment for a patient presenting with tooth wear (TW)
- the suggested protocols for performing an occlusal examination (inclusive of the extra-oral components as well as the intra-oral determinants)
- definitions of the key terms, including a description of the various mandibular positions that are commonly referred to.

This chapter focuses on the more pragmatic elements of clinical occlusion when planning to provide restorative care, with the overall aim of attaining predictability with a functional outcome.

The following topics are addressed:

- The concept of the *ideal occlusion.*
- The fabrication of *appropriate study casts and records to enable occlusal analysis.*
- How and when to take a *conformative approach* to restorative care provision.
- How and when to adopt a *reorganised approach* towards restorative rehabilitation (including cases that require an increase in the occlusal vertical dimension [OVD]).
- The placement of restorations in the *supra-occlusal position, relative axial tooth movement* and the *Dahl phenomenon.*

5.2   The Concept of the Ideal Occlusion

It is perhaps relevant at the outset to draw a distinction between the concept of the *ideal occlusal scheme* and that of a *correct occlusal scheme.*[1] According Davies et al.[2] an occlusal scheme may be described at three levels:

Practical Procedures in the Management of Tooth Wear, First Edition. Subir Banerji, Shamir Mehta, Niek Opdam and Bas Loomans.
© 2020 John Wiley & Sons Ltd. Published 2020 by John Wiley & Sons Ltd.
Companion website: www.wiley.com/go/banerji/toothwear

- tooth
- articulatory system
- patient.

In order to meet the criteria of the ideal occlusal scheme, there is a need for a multitude of precise features at each level to fulfil the overall mechanical and neuromuscular requirements. These features are listed in Table 5.1. It should be noted, however, that much of the information on this ideological concept is based on clinical opinion.

In contrast, an *incorrect occlusal scheme* can be considered to be one that at the time of carrying out the examination is suggestive of the presence of occlusal dysfunction on the basis of the presenting clinical signs and symptoms. Such signs and symptoms may include:[2]

- temporomandibular joint (TMJ) dysfunction/disorders
- occlusal trauma
- recurrent tooth and/or restoration fractures
- hypersensitivity and/or excessive tooth surface loss.

However, it is very common to encounter patients who do not have any of the above signs or indeed the presence of an ideal occlusal scheme (as shown in Table 5.1), and so it may be inappropriate to diagnose the presence of an *incorrect occlusal scheme*. Under such circumstances, whilst a patient may have signs of some degree of TW and the lack of an ideal occlusal scheme, caution needs to be exercised in diagnosing the presence of an erroneous occlusal scheme, and thus the temptation to prescribe invasive treatment(s) as an attempt to attain the mechanical ideal.

From a pragmatic perspective, the concept of a *mutually protected occlusal scheme* (MPO)[3] is often applied by many practitioners when considering

Table 5.1 The features of an ideal occlusal scheme

---

a. At the tooth level

- Multiple simultaneous contacts
- No cuspal incline contacts
- Occlusal contacts that are congruent with the long axis of the tooth
- Smooth and, where possible, shallow contacts during mandibular guidance

b. At the articulatory system level

- Centric occlusion occurring in CR
- Freedom in centric occlusion
- The absence of any posterior interference during dynamic movements, with anterior guidance being provided at the front of the mouth

c. At the patient level

- An occlusal scheme that fits into the neuromuscular tolerances of the patient at that point of time in their life

---

Source: adapted from Davies et al.[2]

restorative rehabilitation, or indeed as a baseline to indicate mechanical stability. The existence of the MPO scheme implies the following:

- In the inter-cuspal position (ICP), the posterior teeth are axially loaded with light occlusal contact present at the anterior teeth, with the posterior teeth effectively protecting the anterior teeth from excessive occlusal loading.[4]
- During dynamic mandibular movements (protrusive as well as lateral excursive), the anterior sextants (including all six anterior pairs of teeth) provide guidance culminating in the separation (*disclusion*) and protection of the posterior teeth from unwanted non-axially directed forces.[3,5]
- At the end of the chewing stroke, only the posterior teeth come into contact, providing the stops for vertical closure and returning the mandible back to the ICP.[5]
- Centric relation (CR) is co-incident with the ICP.[5]

Additional features that may be desirable in a functional occlusion include:

- bilateral contact between the posterior teeth in the retruded contact position (RCP)[6]
- stable stops on all teeth of equal intensity when the condyles are in CR
- an RCP to ICP slide of no more than 1 mm without any lateral deviation[4]
- shared/even occlusal contacts during anterior guidance/protrusive movements with the anterior guidance being in harmony with the border movements of the envelope of function
- canine guided/canine protected occlusion, which is a form of mutually protected articulation whereby the vertical and horizontal overlap of the antagonistic canine teeth ensures posterior disclusion during lateral excursive movements, with planned *group function* on the loss of canine guidance (or where the canine tooth may be unsuitable as a guiding unit) and the *absence of any working or non-working side occlusal interferences* during the undertaking of a lateral excursive movement.

Canine guided occlusion is relatively easier to accomplish from a technical/ clinical perspective when undertaking restorative rehabilitation (as a means of providing lateral guidance) when compared with the scenario of mandibular guidance being provided by a number of posterior teeth on the working side (*group function*), especially when aiming to ensure that working side and non-working side interferences on lateral excursion are duly avoided.[7] Indeed, canine teeth (of good health, form, and bone support) are suited to the role of absorbing occlusal forces on the basis of:

- their favourable crown-to-root ratio
- root morphology (with a relatively longer root offering a relatively superior root surface area with relatively greater levels of periodontal ligament attachment and periodontal proprioceptors)[7]
- the anatomical form of a typical canine clinical crown, often presenting with a concave palatal surface, suggested to be ideally suited to guiding movement of the mandible during dynamic movements[7]
- their position in the arch as a *corner stone* with increased bony support

- their favourable distance from the *fulcrum*, i.e. TMJ, thereby helping to resist unwanted levering forces that may be encountered as the distance between the point where the load is applied and the fulcrum reduces.

However, it should be noted that there is no substantial evidence to support the notion of a canine guided occlusion being superior to any other form of occlusal scheme (such as that of group function).[8]

It has been suggested by Eliyas and Martin[7] that in relation to the management of a worn dentition of a dentate patient, a mutually protective occlusion or a canine protected occlusion should be considered as an appropriate and desirable end point. The manner by which the above features can be predictably incorporated into a patient's occlusal scheme when undertaking the restorative rehabilitation of a severely worn dentition is discussed in this chapter, as well as in Chapters 8, 9 and 12 to 14.

5.3 The Fabrication of Appropriate Study Casts and Records to Enable Occlusal Analysis

5.3.1 Study Casts, Impression Taking, and Articulator Selection

The role of accurate and high-quality study casts when planning the restorative rehabilitation of worn dentition cannot be overemphasised. They permit the following:[9]

- an assessment of the occlusion in the absence of soft tissue/muscular interferences
- further analysis of the static and dynamic features of the patient's occlusal scheme
- planning restorative care during provision and design of restorations and/or dental prostheses.

In order to ensure accuracy of the study casts, impressions should be taken using *rigid impression trays* such as metal rimlock trays or a custom tray (Figure 5.1). Although alginate can be used as a suitable impression material (Figure 5.2), it is preferable to use a high-quality, dimensionally accurate form of alginate or an appropriate polyvinyl silicone (PVS) based material. In either case, it is important to ensure that the manufacturer's instructions are carefully followed in relation to the dispensing, mixing and clinical application of the material, impression decontamination, storage and the casting of the impressions taken. Whilst the use of a silicone material will also allow the pouring of subsequent/duplicate casts (without the need to use duplication techniques), when a more rigid material such as silicone is being used, undercuts must be appropriately blocked out and the presence of a sufficient amount of space ensured between the anatomical structures and the inner surface of the tray to help avoid the impression material and tray from being locked into the patient's mouth.

Vacuum-mixed type III gypsum stone should be used to pour the impressions.[10] On receipt of the casts, they should be inspected for the absence of any obvious distortions (which may be noticeable on the verification of the individual casts and/or on simple hand-articulation assuming that the ICP is stable and readily identifiable). Any marked defects (such as from the casting of airblows and/or heel contacts) should be carefully eased away. However, should this process result in an erroneous occlusal recording, new impressions should be taken. Sometimes, an error with the casts may not be noticed until the process of attempting to fit the cast to an appropriate type of occlusal record (taken using a relatively rigid and accurate material) such as those used on the bite fork when taking a facebow record or an inter-occlusal record, as discussed further below.[10]

There is a diverse variety of *dental articulators* available in the market place.[11] When planning care for a patient often involving complex changes to the existing occlusal scheme, there is a need to study, document, and ultimately copy the dynamic movements of the mandible in the extra-oral environment (as well as reasonably possible). For this purpose, the use of an *arcon* (where the condylar elements are positioned on the lower member of the articulator, akin to the anatomical arrangement, as opposed to a non-arcon form of device) *semi-adjustable articulator* is generally considered appropriate[4] (especially in the general dental practice setting). The latter will permit the programming of the articulator to enable the setting of the *condylar guidance angle, Bennet angle* (progressive side shift), and *immediate side shift* (Bennet movement) using the lateral and protrusive occlusal records, which are particularly relevant when planning the morphology of any posterior restorations.

5.3.2 The Facebow Record

The *facebow* recording is often the first procedure undertaken when the mounting study casts onto a (semi-adjustable) dental articulator. The facebow (also referred to as a *hingebow*) is a rigid but adjustable device that relates the maxillary occlusal surface to an *anatomical reference point*.[12] The primary purpose of the facebow record is to permit mounting of the maxillary cast on the articulator. In addition, the facebow also provides a guide to the width between the condyles, referred to as the *inter-condylar width*, which has further practical significance in relation to the morphology of the posterior restorations (should they be part of the treatment plan).

Typically, two reference points are chosen when attaining a facebow record: a *posterior reference point*, usually the terminal hinge axis, which is an imaginary line that runs between the heads of the mandibular condyles (that relates to the condylar elements of the articulator), and a second, more *anterior reference point*. The latter may vary between occlusal apparatus. Both anterior and posterior reference points should be replicable during further subsequent appointments. Typical anterior reference points include *Nasion or the inner canthus of the eye*.

Facebows generally fall into the category of being either arbitrary or kinematic.[5] *Arbitrary facebows* are less accurate in the manner in which they relate to the terminal hinge axis. They are, however, suitable for most routine restorative dental procedures. Arbitrary facebows effectively approximate the position of the *terminal hinge axis* typically to the position of the external auditory meatus (which is erroneous by definition). Facebows that utilise the external auditory meatus as the reference point are commonly referred to as *earbows*.

In contrast, the use of a *kinematic facebow* requires the terminal hinge axis to be more accurately determined, which may be more relevant where there is a need to copy the precise opening and closing movements of the mandible on the dental articulator, such as for a complex restorative reconstruction involving an alteration of the existing vertical and horizontal occlusal relations.

The *facebow fork* or *bite fork* is an item of equipment that is used to record the maxillary occlusal surfaces using a variety of different media/materials. These materials should offer dimensional stability, a suitable working time, and ease of use. Typically the applied recording materials include Brown Impression Compound, Greenstick, PVS bite registration materials (such as Stonebite [Dreve Dentamid GmbH, Germany] and Blue Mousee [Parkell Inc., USA]) or extra hard wax, such as Moyco Beauty wax (Moyco Industries, USA).

The record obtained using the bite fork is then inserted into the facebow, thus permitting the attainment of the registration required.

The procedure for taking a facebow record described below relates to the use of the *Denar Mark II System* (Whipmix, KY, USA), utilising the *Denar Slidematic facebow*.[13] This is an example of an arbitrary facebow where the articulator is of the arcon semi-adjustable variety. This system is widely used in clinical practice internationally and most laboratories and dental technicians are familiar with it.

The facebow recording procedure usually starts by using the *reference point indicator* in the Denar Slidematic facebow kit, whereby the anterior reference point for facebow transfer is identified and marked up. This should be 43 mm from the patient's incisal edge of either the right central or lateral incisor towards the inner canthus (corner) of their right eye. For an edentulous patient the lower border of the upper lip at rest is used. There may also be an indication to measure and record the distance between this reference point and the inner canthus of their right eye, in the event that the anterior reference point may be lost through a dental extraction or restorative intervention of one of the reference incisor teeth.

The chosen material for recording the occlusal surface of the maxillary arch should then be applied onto the correct surface of the bite fork. When using a thermoplastic material such as wax or an impression compound, the temperature of the material should be carefully checked to avoid unwanted scalding of the patient's lips and face.

The bite fork is inserted into the patient's mouth and carefully centred over the maxillary cusp tips, lightly compressing it in order to attain an impression. Some protocols advocate instructing the patient to bite down gently into the recording medium. The index ring on the fork should ideally line up with the patient's midline (as shown by the accompanying video-graphic presentation). The overall objective (according to the manufacturer) is to produce a 'slight impression' of the cusp tips, primarily avoiding fossae.[13] It is not essential to record every cusp; the level of detail required should be enough to permit the seating of an accurate maxillary cast in a stable manner. A record that is very shallow will not permit accurate and reproducible seating of the cast. In contrast, a record that is too deep will not permit accurate repositioning, as the casts are not a precise duplication of the teeth.

When using a wax-based material or impression compound (such as Brown Impression Compound or Greenstick Composition, Kerr, USA), cooling of the material using a three-in-one air gun is advisable, followed by the subsequent removal of the record from the patient's mouth; the registration material may then be chilled under cold water. Clearly, this stage will not be necessary when using PVS materials. The record should then be carefully assessed and re-seated to assess for distortion and stability, which may be indicated by the presence of a rocking motion when the bite fork is re-positioned and supported by the index fingers on either side of the bite fork. Where the record may reveal unwanted details such as pits and fissures, the recording medium should be carefully trimmed prior to re-seating the model using a scalpel. If there are any perforations through the registration medium (with metal display), the cast will not seat accurately. Under such circumstances, a new record needs to be taken.

It is good practice to have the maxillary cast at the operator's disposal prior to the facebow recording. This will allow the clinician to check that the cast seats accurately and positively into the record in the bite fork, whilst concomitantly verifying the accuracy of the study cast. In the event of an error, it is advisable to take new impressions. Patel and Alani[10] described the use of a separate bite fork to take a record of the mandibular arch to verify the accuracy of this cast.

For the next stage, some level of patient assistance is required. With the bite fork in situ, a request should be made for the patient to place their thumbs on either under-side of the bite fork or support the fork using a pair of cotton wool rolls placed against the occlusal surfaces of the lower posterior teeth. The patient should then be instructed to gently bite down.

The *reference pin* should be fastened to the underside of the facebow, and all of the toggles and clamps on the Denar Slidematic facebow subsequently loosened. The clamp marked 2 should then be slid over the protruding end of the bite fork towards the patient's face. The clamp should be positioned over the shaft on the right side of the patient. Each of the *calliper ends* are then placed into the patient's external auditory opening (similar to a stethoscope). It can be helpful to have a dental assistant guide the positioning of the calliper end on the side that the operator is facing away from. Where the choice is taken to use cotton wool roll to help support the fork in situ, the patient may be requested to position the earpieces themselves, particularly if placement appears to be proving to be difficult and/or uncomfortable, typically, for instance, where the ears are at slightly different levels.

The anterior reference pointer should now be carefully released and positioned so that it points towards the anterior reference point marked earlier. The facebow is then slid upwards or downwards so that the tip of the reference pointer contacts the reference point; at this point the bow will be horizontal to the Frankfort plane. The screw on clamp 1 should then be tightened (the vertical reference pin), whilst the screw on clamp 2 serves as the horizontal reference pin. At this point, the numbers 1 and 2 on the clamps should be facing in the direction of the operator. The toggles and clamps should next be tightened until the recording apparatus is secure (Figure 5.3).

On the superior surface of the facebow is a scale. It is relevant to make a note of this measurement, which serves as an indication to the *inter-condylar width*. This can also be used to position the condylar pillars of the articulator.

Finally, the calliper screw should be slackened, the facebow carefully removed from the patient's ears, and the entire device taken out of the patient's mouth and appropriately disinfected. The facebow and bite fork assembly can be separated and carefully transported.

The assembly is then transferred to the articulator (in part or whole) depending on the apparatus being used. The maxillary cast is positioned onto the occlusal record, which is related to the terminal hinge axis on the articulator, and the cast attached to a mounting plate on the articulator using a suitable mounting stone/plaster.

5.3.3   The Taking of Inter-occlusal Records

Accurate inter-occlusal records of the selected variety can be used to relate the occlusal surfaces of mandibular cast to those of the maxillary cast, thereby permitting the mounting of a set of casts against each other on the articulator. Inter-occlusal records generally take the form of:

- Inter-cuspal position records
- CR records
- lateral/protrusive records.

The *inter-cuspal record* by definition records the position where the antagonistic occlusal surfaces are maximally meshed together. The *CR record*, however, aims to record the relationship of the mandibular arch to that of the maxillary arch when the condyles are seated in their most *anterior-superior positions* in the glenoid fossae. In the latter position (as discussed in Chapter 4), the opening and closing movements of the mandible take place in a rotational manner (as opposed to translation) for the first few millimetres and correspond to rotational movements occurring at the dental articulator's condylar housing.

Lateral excursive and/or protrusive mandibular records may also be taken in conjunction with the CR record in order to programme the condylar guides on the articulator, which would relate to the anatomical limits of the movements of the condyles in their glenoid fossae.

5.3.3.1   The Intercuspal Record

An inter-cuspal record is generally taken when mounting a set of working casts where the occlusal scheme is stable, often where relatively simple restorations are being considered, hence a need to conform to the existing occlusal scheme. The use of casts mounted in CR for this purpose may culminate in undesirable occlusal interference.

For a dentate patient where the occlusal surfaces inter-relate in a manner where the inter-cuspal position is readily determined, an inter-cuspal record may be attained by placing a suitable quantity of recording material such as PVS-based bite registration paste onto a dried occlusal surface (such as that of a tooth preparation) or bilaterally across the posterior occluding surfaces. Other materials such as Moyco Beauty wax or cold cured acrylic resins may also be used, for example Duralay (Reliance Dental Manufacturing Co. Worth, Illinois, USA) Palavit G (Kulzer) or Trim (Bosworth, USA). However, where possible the record should be as close to *zero thickness* in key areas.

Once the chosen recording material has been placed evenly onto the patient's occlusal surface, the patient should be asked to bring their teeth together into the position of best fit, a process that can sometimes prove difficult for some patients. Once set, the record is carefully removed and used to mount the casts on the articulator.

The accuracy of the mounting can be determined by using ultra-thin foil articulating paper. The holding contacts identified intra-orally should be congruent with those on the dental casts (Figure 5.4). If they are not, this may be indicative of an error. As discussed above, it is important to appraise the casts for any casting nodules or incorrectly trimmed models, especially in the heel areas.

For partially dentate patients, there may be a need to fabricate a wax occlusal rim, ideally supported by an acrylic base plate.

5.3.3.2 The CR Record

The CR record (unlike the inter-cuspal record) is attained *regardless of any given position of tooth contact.* The CR record is often referred to as being a *fixed and reproducible record* in the literature; fixed in this context is in reference to a fixed anatomical position (independent of the occlusal surfaces) that is reproducible between the patient's condyles and the condylar housing of the dental articulator (where rotational movements of the condyles will take place against the corresponding articular eminences).

The CR record is advocated when fabricating study casts, thereby permitting the evaluation of the RCP, also sometimes referred to as the centric relation contact position (CRCP), the retruded axis position (RAP) or terminal hinge position (THP), which is the first point of tooth contact whilst the mandible is in CR. Evaluation of the RCP may otherwise be very difficult in the presence of the soft tissues and protective neuromuscular reflexes of the patient.

Approximately 90% of patients have a slide between RCP and ICP (with ICP being anterior and superior to CR by 1.25 mm ±1.0 mm);[14] casts mounted in CR can readily elucidate this feature if present. Any *premature tooth contacts*, also termed *deflective contacts* (that will guide the patient's mandible from CRCP to ICP) can be noted at this stage as well as the need for any occlusal correction determined (prior to embarking upon complex prosthodontics treatment plans).

For patients with *pathological TW* (especially when active restorative intervention is likely), the identification of RCP may be helpful for the following reasons:

- CR is a mandibular position that is independent of tooth contact (and has been found to be reproducible within 0.08 mm due to the non-elastic nature of the TMJ capsule and associated capsular ligaments).[15] It would seem sensible to apply this position when undertaking complex occlusal rehabilitation in order to provide a reproducible reference point not only between the arches (including cases where an increase in the OVD is planned), but one which also serves as a fixed position between the patient and the dental articulator that can be replicated. At this position the movement of the condyles is a simple hinge movement that can then be transferred onto the articulator as this hinge movement would be the first movement here also.

- The discrepancy between RCP and ICP may result in a level of inter-occlusal clearance (in either the vertical or horizontal dimension) that may be utilised to place restorative materials when reorganising the occlusion and help to alleviate the need to increase the occlusal dimension or the need for subtractive tooth preparation to accommodate future restorations, as discussed further below and in Chapters 9 and 10.
- CR could also be chosen for the construction of full coverage occlusal splints, which may be used for the management of parafunctional habits (that may lead to TW), for the protection of heavily restored dentitions, and also to plan restorative rehabilitation of patients with generalised TW, whereby a temporary, removable ideal occlusal scheme (which represents the desired end point of the restorative process) is tried out for tolerance in an minimally invasive manner. The role of occlusal splints for the management of TW is discussed in depth in Chapter 7.

A CR record may also be contemplated where the tooth being restored by the means of an indirect restoration is the first point of tooth contact in CR, either to copy this onto the definitive restoration or as a means of evaluating a possible change in the RCP onto a tooth which may be suboptimal for the process of further occlusal loading.

In order to attain a *record of CR*, there is the need to *locate CR*. This is not always a straightforward matter, however, often as a result of the presence of protective neuromuscular reflexes (which may be encountered amongst patients with parafunctional habits) as well the level of occlusal disharmony present.[10] Other factors that have been described by Wilson and Banerjee[16] to influence the ease with which CR may be located (and recorded) include:

- the level of patient (cooperativity, their understanding of the process, their state of relaxation, and their spatial position)
- the operator's level of experience and training
- the registration material and recording method used
- the time of the recording
- guidance of the mandible
- neuromuscular conditioning
- record handling and storage.

A number of *operator-guided techniques* for the manual manipulation of the condyles (for dentate patients) into the desired position for recording the CR have been described in the literature, including:[16]

- the chin-point guidance method
- the three-finger chin-point guidance method
- the power centric registration method
- the bimanual manipulation method.

The technique of *bimanual manipulation*, as described by Dawson,[17] is often advocated in the literature and warrants further appraisal. With this approach, the patient should be seated in the dental chair in a supine position with the operator seated directly behind. The operator's fifth and fourth fingers of each hand should be placed behind the angle of the mandible and in front of the angle, respectively, to allow the condyles to be directed antero-superiorly. The third fingers are placed on the inferior border of the mandible, the index fingers positioned submentally in the midline, and the thumbs placed laterally to the symphysis.[16,17]

The patient should then be instructed to relax their jaw and allow the operator to control the jaw movements. The mandible should be slowly and gently arced upwards and downwards with minimal force. The upward movement should be gradually increased until the first point of contact is reached. If undertaken correctly, the mandible will be hinged along its retruded arc of closure. It may be possible to palpate this portion of the condyle by placing a finger into the patient's external auditory meatus. It is important, however, to avoid the use of a forceful action that will inadvertently push the mandible backwards towards a downward transalatory movement, culminating in an erroneous record and well as patient discomfort (resulting in resistance to the applied load).[16]

It is also worthwhile asking the patient if they may be aware of the side of their jaw where the first point of tooth contact occurs in CR. The patient should then be requested to squeeze their teeth together, with the operator noting the direction of the slide of the jaw into ICP.[12] The first point of tooth contact can be marked up, ideally using two different colours of GHM occlusal indicating paper (Hanel GHM Dental, Germany) and Shimstock foil (supported using either Millers forceps or Artery forceps) to mark up the slide from RCP to ICP.[10]

To assist with more challenging cases where these techniques prove ineffective in locating CR, the use of an *anterior de-programming device* may prove helpful. The latter can overcome the neuromuscular reflexes, which are initiated by tooth contact, by causing tooth separation and providing an anterior reference point/stop to help stabilise the mandible during the act of taking the record.[16] For this purpose, the patient can be instructed to bite on some *cotton wool rolls*, ensuring that all the teeth are separated (by a minimal distance that permits the effective use of the recording medium) or a set of *wooden spatulas* (*tongue blade method*), where it has been suggested that the teeth should be discluded for a period of 10–20 minutes (to allow the proprioceptive input to be lost) prior to taking the registration.[16]

Commercially available products may provide a better option for the above purpose. An example of a commonly used device is the *Leaf Gauge* (Huffman Dental Products LLC, OH, USA) as depicted by Figure 5.5. The Leaf Gauge is composed of thin plastic strips of 0.1 mm width that are placed in the anterior region; further layers are sequentially added until there is evidence of posterior tooth separation when the patient bites down lightly. Once CR has been located, occlusal stops can be prepared using direct resin composite to record and relocate this position. This technique is frequently used by the authors.

For some patients, however, it may still remain difficult to locate CR. Under such circumstances it is appropriate to fabricate an anterior de-programming device, such as a *Lucia Jig*.

The Lucia Jig is effectively an anterior bite plane/platform deprogrammer, first described by Lucia in 1964, traditionally constructed using cold cured acrylic resins (such as Duralay, Palavit G or Trim, Bosworth). An example is shown in Figure 5.6a; in this case, the Jig was prepared prior to patient arrival, where extra-oral fabrication on a cast (as in this case) can avoid the polymerisation exotherm that can prove unpleasant for some patients when the device is fabricated intra-orally.

The Jig should be sculpted such that it just covers the palatal soft tissues and has a slope of approximately 40–60°.[16] An additional merit of the Jig in improving the efficacy of the device in determining CR is by enabling the undertaking of a *gothic-arch tracing*. The patient is advised to make lateral excursive and protrusive movements with the Lucia Jig in situ and a piece of articulating paper is imposed between the jig and the mandibular incisor teeth. A point is selected from the lower dentition to form the pattern on the Jig (by removing the influence of the other teeth by either undertaking selective adjustment of the Jig or placing a small stylus made from adding a small amount of flowable resin composite to one of the lower incisor teeth, ensuring the removal of the stylus prior to discharging of the patient). It would be hoped that ultimately a tracing could be produced on the Jig that will result in a gothic arch pattern with the apex of the arch indicating the retruded mandibular relaxation, as seen in Figure 5.6.

Other techniques that have been described by Wilson and Banerjee to help locate CR include:[16]

- the use of digital pantograph machines
- the use of an electric jaw muscle stimulating device to assist with the attainment of muscle relaxation, the *Myo-monitor*.

For patients who continue to fail to permit manipulation of the mandible after having placed the jig in situ for more than 30 minutes, the use of an appropriate form of full coverage acrylic based *occlusal stabilisation splint* as discussed in Chapter 7 may be indicated.

Having located CR, there is of course a need to record it. Commonly used materials for this purpose are PVS-based bite registration pastes or extra hard dental wax such as Moyco Beauty wax. When planning to use the latter form of material (*wax record*) it is helpful to prepare the inter-occlusal records prior to the patient's arrival. For such records, the outline of should extend approximately 5 mm beyond the buccal cusp tips and use a minimum of two sheets of wax sealed together. Some operators choose to support the wax record with a section of shellac placed between the two layers.

Where the use of a Lucia Jig (or an alternative device) may be required, a relief can be cut into the anterior portion of the wax record to permit concurrent placement of both the record and the jig. Upon patient arrival, the wax record should be re-softened and placed over the maxillary occluding surfaces. The record should be lightly pressed against the cusp tips to produce shallow indentations, and the patient's mandible subsequently guided into CR to develop shallow indentations of the mandibular teeth cusps. The wax record should then be cooled using a three-in-one air and water gun. On removal, the record should be carefully inspected and verified for the absence of any signs of perforation. The record should be chilled using cold water and re-positioned it to verify the accuracy of the record. Some operators choose to use a material such as Temp Bond (Kerr, Orange, CA, USA) to refine the occlusal contacts.

The fit of the CR record should next be checked on the dental casts, avoiding the temptation to squeeze the record to make it fit. An obvious drawback to the use of a thermoplastic material such as wax is distortion on cooling. To help indicate the presence of possible unwanted distortion on cooling and/or transfer to the dental laboratory, the application of a stripe of zinc oxide eugenol paste such as Temp-Bond across a portion of the record may be helpful; cracking of this in due course may be indicative of unwanted distortion.

For a patient who may be partially dentate or edentulous, wax rims mounted on a stable (ideally rigid) base plate will be needed, which should be placed accurately onto the casts.

The CR record may then be used to mount the maxillary cast against the mandibular cast, which in turn can be attached to the lower member of the articulator. Where possible, the lower cast should be mounted as soon as possible to avoid the risk of deformation; indeed, many clinicians carry out this phase immediately after taking the record in the operatory.[10]

5.3.3.3 Lateral and Protrusive Records

There appears to be a lack of clarity in the manner by which lateral and protrusive occlusal records are taken clinically. Whilst some advocate the manipulation of the patient's dentition into one whereby the incisor teeth and canine teeth meet at an edge-to-edge location (representative of the protrusive position and lateral excursion, respectively), in the view of the authors, given that these records represent condylar movement within the glenoid fossa, the record should be taken independent of the teeth.

The technical execution would involve the preparation of a wax-record analogous to the one described above for the recording of CR with an additional layer of wax on the working side (to take account of the extra level of tooth separation when making dynamic movements).[5] The operator can help the patient guide their mandible into excursive and protrusive movements within the likely envelope of function (beyond which the patient may express discomfort).

The technique preferred by the authors involves having the patient supine in a comfortable position and with the mandible relaxed. The mandible is then guided in lateral excursion without any influence of the dentition. While supporting the mandible in the lateral position some composite can be used in the canine region on the side of the excursion to locate this position (without any preparation of the enamel with etching or bonding agents) with the existing teeth not in contact. Subsequently, using the set composite as a guide, the patient can be asked to close and a recording material such as softened beauty wax placed, which would then record this open lateral position of the mandible. The process is repeated on the contralateral side. These left and right lateral records can also be used to determine the condylar guidance angle during protrusion of the mandible. The video resource accompanying this chapter illustrates the technique on a patient.

As part of the accompanying graphical presentation, the use of a technique involving the placement of a Leaf Gauge and/or Lucia Jig is shown, which some clinicians may find helpful in attaining consistency when taking these records, which has been reported to be challenging.[3]

Finally, it is important to verify the *accuracy of the mounting process*. This is typically done by comparing the clinical observations to those seen on the mounted casts using Shimstock bite foil (which should have a thickness of 8 μm). In the event of disparity, there may be a need to re-check the occlusal scheme clinically, and if required to repeat the process of taking the CR record followed by remounting of the mandibular cast. Some authors indeed advocate the taking of multiple (three to five) CR records to permit comparison and allow the mounting of the record they feel most appropriate.[10]

5.4   How and When to Take the Conformative Approach to Restorative Rehabilitation

The *conformative* approach to the restorative rehabilitation of a worn dentition involves the provision of restorations to the affected teeth at the pre-existing occlusal scheme without incurring a change in the OVD and the existing ICP.[7] Therefore, a conformative approach is generally *not indicated* in circumstances that may involve:[2,18]

- an increase in the OVD
- severely malpositioned tooth/teeth with unacceptable function and/or aesthetics
- evidence of occlusal dysfunction, including signs of recurrently failure, de-bonding or fracture of existing restorations due to an underlying occlusal cause
- signs of trauma from the occlusion (soft tissue or periodontal)
- a recurrence of TMJ disorders that may have relapsed following a period of successful occlusal splint therapy.

In the case of worn dentition, given that *dento-alveolar compensation* often follows the loss of coronal tissue from the affected surfaces to maintain the functional merits of the masticatory system[19] (as discussed further in Section 5.7), thereby maintaining antagonistic units in contact, seldom will inter-occlusal clearance be required to accommodate a dental material that would be placed at/on the worn tooth/tooth surfaces to restore the presenting pathology. Consequently, there is a need to provide the desired inter-occlusal clearance. This may be achieved by either:

1) placing the restoration in a *supra-occlusal position* (often using minimally invasive techniques), involving either a planned increase in the OVD, and/or adopting a re-organised approach (utilising any space that may be present between RCP and ICP)

   or

2) undertaking *subtractive* tooth preparation(s) to create the required space (which in the case of worn dentition may also require pre-restorative procedures such a crown lengthening, as discussed further in Chapter 14).

Whilst the second approach may permit the application of a conformative protocol, in general it is not advocated as the initial treatment style of choice,[20] especially given the recent advances in adhesive dentistry, clinical occlusion, the available dental materials, and, of course, the established biological consequences of undertaking invasive tooth preparations (especially amongst teeth that in some cases have sustained severe loss of tooth tissue), as discussed at length in Chapter 10.

A conformative approach is therefore unlikely to be used in the restorative rehabilitation of worn dentition except in the following cases:

- In the presence of *localised TW*, where the required inter-occlusal clearance is available in the ICP (as in the case of the affected tooth having no antagonistic contact, as may be seen with an 'open bite' or where the rate of wear exceeds the rate of dento-alveolar compensation) and presenting ICP is considered to be otherwise stable.
- In the case of *localised TW*, where the placement of a restoration in supra-occlusion is not indicated due to unfavourable circumstances or a failure to gain consent, resulting in the need for a subtractive approach (assuming the tooth is not involved as the first point of contact in CR).
- In the case of *generalised TW*, where space is not present as a result of the lack of discrepancy between RCP and ICP, and a physiological freeway space of 2–4 mm is maintained (for further details refer to Chapter 13).
- In cases of minor wear, where restorative intervention may be indicated.

From a practical perspective, when a conformative approach is to be taken it is imperative to leave sufficient reference points to make sure that the new restorations do indeed conform to the existing occlusal scheme.

Accordingly, a set of study casts should be fabricated, a facebow record taken and if necessary a record of the ICP as well as lateral and protrusive records (as per Section 5.3.3.3), and the casts suitably mounted on a semi-adjustable articulator. In order to maintain reference points, it may be sensible to prepare alternative teeth on different visits (where multiple restorations are being prescribed) and/or obtain an ICP record immediately following the preparation of some teeth by interposing a dimensionally stable registration medium (as an appropriate form of PVS bite registration material or a cold cured acrylic) between the opposing occluding surfaces in the ICP. The latter can then be used to mount the working cast against the opposing pre-mounted study cast.

Where the affected tooth/teeth may be involved in providing mandibular guidance, a *customised incisal guidance table* (also sometimes referred to as an anterior guidance table or incisal bite table[4]) can be prepared to 'copy' the occlusal prescription and features of the guiding surfaces, thereby preserving the desired dynamic occlusal scheme.[2] The technical stages are as follows:

a) *Pre-definitive restoration casts* should be correctly mounted on a semi-adjustable articulator, as described above.
b) The incisal pin of the articulator should then be raised by approximately 2 mm.
c) The tip of the incisal pin should be lightly coated in petroleum jelly (to act as a separator).
d) An appropriate quantity of cold-cured acrylic should be mixed according to the manufacturer's instructions, and when at the doughy stage the material should be transferred to the incisal guidance table.
e) Whilst the acrylic material is still setting, the tip of the incisal pin should be transcribed through the material by moving the upper member of the articulator backwards and from side to side, thereby guiding the incisors though

simulated excursive and protrusive movements; in this way, a record will have been made of the articulator during dynamic movements.

f) Once set, it is important to verify that the incisal pin has formed a patent contact with the registration material (thereby ensuring that the ICP has been maintained). This can be checked using a section of Shimstock articulating foil.

g) The table can be carefully trimmed to remove any excess, without compromising the record.

h) The working cast can now be mounted against the antagonistic pre-existing cast (using an inter-cuspal record if necessary).

i) The customised incisal guidance table (Figure 5.7) can be used to fabricate the definitive restoration, using the record of the pre-restorative envelope of mandibular movement to determine the desirable crown height, length, and anatomy of the guiding surfaces.[2] In an analogous manner, it is important to ensure that the incisal pin remains in contact with the guidance table in the appropriate manner, which can be verified using Shimstock foil as well as GHM articulating paper.

5.5   How and When to Adopt a Reorganised Approach

According to Eliyas and Martin,[7] a reorganised approach 'requires the restoration of worn teeth in CR with an increase in OVD'. Further to Section 5.4, the reorganised approach to the restorative rehabilitation of a patient with TW is likely to be commonly prescribed and may range from the more relatively simple task of restoration of canine guidance to more demanding cases of full mouth rehabilitation; for further details refer to Chapters 10 and 14, respectively.

The protocol for undertaking a reorganised approach for the restorative rehabilitation of a patient with TW in outline involves the following:

1) The mounting of a set of casts using the CR record, concomitantly programming the articulator settings using a set of appropriate lateral and protrusive inter-occlusal records.

2) The scale of the difference between RCP and ICP will become readily apparent from the mounted casts; for some patients the space between these positions will indeed be sufficient to allow restorative intervention. Indeed, in patients with severe TW, often presenting with the loss of posterior cusp tips and a wearing/ failing anterior guidance, there is a tendency for the condyle to gradually anteriorly slide forward. Thus, locating CR can give the effect of *distalising the mandible*; the resultant space that may be gained can prove invaluable during restorative rehabilitation.[16]

3) In other cases there will be a need to plan an increase in the OVD (by raising the pin on the articulator) in order to fulfil the requirements of the dental material to perform optimally, fulfil the functional needs, and meet the aesthetic requirements of the patient (whilst respecting the limitations of the functional envelope). It has been suggested that the increase in vertical height can be up to 20–25 mm (taken between fixed reference points between antagonistic anterior teeth) in dentate patients, where the condyles remain in the desired position when recording CR, displaying rotation movement only around the terminal hinge axis.[7]

4) Having determined the occlusal prescription (as well as establishing the aesthetic prescription, as detailed in Chapter 9), a diagnostic wax up may be prepared accordingly to fulfil the aesthetic requirements and provide the *ideal occlusal scheme* as discussed in Section 5.2 above; in summary providing a *mutually protective occlusion* or *canine occlusal scheme.*

5) Next, it is important to verify the patient's *acceptance of the planned occlusal scheme.* Where possible this should be accomplished by using a minimally invasive approach that allows ease of adjustment and, ideally, full reversal.[21] Historically, in the case of patient requiring a full mouth reconstructing (*displaying generalised TW*) the latter has been accomplished by the use of an *occlusal stabilisation splint* (see Chapter 7), which provides a *temporary, removable ideal occlusal scheme (at the desired OVD).*

6) Splint compliance can, however, be problematic. Consequently, there has now been a move towards the use of adhesively retained restorations to 'test drive' the occlusal scheme, which can be placed with minimal, irreversible tooth tissue loss. The latter is most often accomplished by taking a PVS index of the occluding surfaces of the diagnostic wax up and using this information to assist/guide the placement of direct resin composite restorations.

7) With the current advances in digital dentistry, the use of CAD/CAM techniques to plan and ultimately fabricate indirect resin restorations may also provide the clinician with an alternative approach to the use of direct restorations, with advantages that are discussed in Chapter 14. In either case, the occlusal splint or resin retained restorations can be readily adjusted either by a process of addition or subtraction of material until the required functional and aesthetic outcomes have been achieved.[21]

8) In the longer term, having established functional stability and aesthetic and functional tolerance, indirect restorations can be predictably provided (which may be more costly and invasive but offer superior aesthetics and mechanical properties) using the *conformative approach* described above.

9) Where the use of conventionally retained crowns/onlays has been planned at the outset (for instance where the use of adhesively retained restorations may not be suitable or the patient has a heavily restored dentition comprising existing crown and bridge work), the use of *provisional restorations* will help to provide a predictable approach (with or without the prior prescription of a full coverage occlusal stabilisation splint, as detailed in Chapter 7).

10) Under such circumstances, the diagnostic wax-up can be duplicated. Using the duplicate cast, a *vacuum formed stent/splint* can be prepared in the laboratory.

11) Following the process of tooth preparation (which can be further guided using indices made from the wax-up to help provide a precision approach to carrying out tooth reduction), the stent/splint can be used to fabricate *custom-direct (chairside based) provisional restorations* using the desired crown and bridge resin. It would be advisable to prepare alternative teeth in order to allow single unit restorations to be provided, with the aim of optimising periodontal health by allowing for the practice of good oral hygiene procedures and also to ascertain the true tolerance as detailed below.

12) Alternatively, the dental technician can undertake tooth preparations on the mounted duplicate casts and fabricate *custom indirect 'shell-type' acrylic based provisional crowns* with the occlusal end point incorporated in these

restorations. The latter shells can then be relined chairside by the addition of a suitable material.

13) Some clinicians, however, prefer to take an impression following the completion of the preparations. The resultant casts can then be mounted using suitable inter-occlusal records in CR, and *custom indirect provisional* restorations fabricated in the laboratory to meet the occlusal ideals and aesthetic prescription. There are, of course, advantages and disadvantages of each of the options listed above; for further information, kindly refer to a reputable textbook in restorative dentistry/ fixed prosthodontics.

14) In either case, the provisional restorations should be tried and adjusted as necessary, either by subtraction or the addition of direct resin composite, until the appropriate occlusal contacts and aesthetics have been developed. The restorations should then be cemented in using a provisional cement. The patient should be periodically reviewed for tolerance and adaptation by assessing the following:
   - The presence of the desired occlusal scheme at the time of appraisal – with mutual protection, ideally with a canine guided occlusion (although this may be challenging in the case of a patient with an anterior open bite, incisal edge to edge or Class III relationship).[4] The ultimate aim, of course, is to achieve posterior disclusion when performing dynamic jaw movements.
   - Whilst it would be optimal to have shared occlusal contact on protrusion between the six pairs of anterior antagonistic teeth, in some cases (such as with lower incisor crowding),[4] this may be very challenging to achieve practically. Therefore, whilst guidance is protrusion should be avoided at one single tooth (especially that of a maxillary lateral incisor), some level of compromise may need to be reached.[4]
   - Recurrent fracture of the provisional restoration(s).
   - Recurrent de-bonding/ loosening.
   - Tooth mobility.
   - Discomfort.
   - Endodontic and periodontal complications.
   - Difficulty with mastication and phonetics.
   - Aesthetic outcome.

15) The provisional restorations may therefore require adjustment as described above until all parties are satisfied. Following an observation period of approximately six to eight weeks, with the patient reporting the lack of any symptoms and signs to suggest a functionally and aesthetically acceptable outcome, the features of provisional restorations may be copied using a conformative approach. Impressions should be taken of the provisional restorations in situ and the *pre-definitive restoration casts mounted in ICP, concomitantly employing the use of a customised incisal guidance table to copy the dynamic prescription that will have been established by the process of using provisional restorations.*

16) Ceramic-based restorations may be tried in at the biscuit stage to allow some adjustments to be made prior to the final glazing process.

17) The definitive restorations may be cemented initially using a temporary cement to allow a further period of appraisal.

In summary, the above protocol would aim to achieve an outcome whereby RCP and ICP would be co-incident. Hopefully, it will now also be apparent that in essence the only clear difference between the conformative approach and the reorganised approach from the point of technical execution, is that the latter requires some additional stages of planning and design before providing the definitive restorations by using a technique to conform to the newly prescribed occlusal scheme that would have been determined by the careful use of techniques that permit adjustment with relative ease.

In relation to the reorganised occlusal scheme, it is worthwhile noting the observations of Celenza,[22] who has shown that the slide from ICP to RCP will re-establish within a period of 2–12 years (possibly due to the effect of condylar remodelling as well as the progressive wear of the restorative materials). This may perhaps challenge the need to be 'absolute' when trying to restore to a precise position, i.e. that of CR. The latter is perhaps further supported by the plethora of possible errors that may occur when trying to accurately located and record CR (including impression taking, casting, taking occlusal records, mounting the casts as per the records attained and the limitations of the design of articulator used), whereby the perceived location of CR may be inaccurate.[8] Indeed, the capacity of the patient to adapt to the changes implemented perhaps has a very important role,[16] which, as discussed below, may to some extent challenge many traditionally held concepts in relation to clinical occlusion.

5.6 The Placement of Dental Restorations in Supra-occlusion: The Dahl Concept

For the majority of patients, TW is accompanied by *dento-alveolar compensation.*[19] This is a form of physiological compensatory mechanism that allows occlusal contacts to be maintained despite the process of tooth tissue loss in order to attempt to preserve the efficacy of the masticatory system. The process of dento-alveolar compensation does, however, lead to the loss of the inter-occlusal space (that would otherwise exist due to the loss of tooth tissue), and thereby presents a technical challenge from a restorative perspective in relation to the provision of space to accommodate the chosen restorative material.

Historically, traditional prosthodontic protocols for the restorative management of TW have involved the need to undertake irreversible tooth reduction in order to create the space required to accommodate conventionally retained crown and onlay restorations/restorative materials. However, it has been well documented that the preparation of teeth to receive full coverage indirect restoration may culminate in not only the irreversible loss of pulp vitality but also the marked loss of coronal volume.[23,24] In the case of a worn dentition, the further loss of tooth tissue may prove to be highly detrimental.

Whilst in some cases of TW the required inter-occlusal clearance can be attained by adopting a reorganised approach towards the rehabilitative process (by utilising the discrepancy between RCP and ICP as discussed above), this approach may unfortunately culminate in several teeth (often teeth unaffected/ relatively unaffected by TW) needing restorations in order to maintain occlusal stability. This will further add to the complexity of care, the longer-term mainte- nance requirements, and the treatment cost. Under such circumstances, where there is a need to avoid subtractive tooth preparations, one possible option may be the placement of restorations in a *supra-occlusal position*, a concept com- monly referred to as the *Dahl concept* or *Dahl phenomenon*. This is now com- monly utilised for restoration in patients presenting with localised TW, as discussed further in Chapters 11 and 12.[25]

In 1975, Dahl et al.[25] reported the use of a removable anterior bite platform, fabricated from cobalt chromium, retained by clasps in the canine and premolar regions to create inter-occlusal space in a patient with TW localised to the ante- rior maxillary segment. The appliance was designed to cover the cingulum rears of the affected teeth and increase the occlusal vertical dimension by around 2–3 mm. The placement of the appliance culminated in posterior teeth disclu- sion; occlusal contacts were only present between the mandibular anterior teeth and the bite platform.

This *Dahl appliance* was prescribed for continual wear for several months until the posterior teeth re-established inter-occlusal contact. Removal of the appliance resulted in an inter-occlusal space between the anterior maxillary and mandibular dentitions, which was subsequently utilised to restore the worn sur- faces without the need for further tooth reduction.

Dahl and Krungstad[26] proceeded to use this device on a series of patients and reported that in most cases re-establishment of occlusal contacts occurred within 4–6 months. It has since been suggested, however, that re-establishment may take up to 18–24 months in some cases.[27]

The actual Dahl concept refers to the *relative axial tooth movement* that is observed to occur when a localised appliance or localised restoration(s) are placed in supra-occlusion and the occlusion re-establishes full arch contacts over a period of time. The concept is thought to occur through a process of controlled *intrusion and extrusion* of the *dento-alveolar segments*.

It was reported by Dahl and Krungstad[26] that the inter-occlusal space created occurs through a process of combined intrusion (40%) and extrusion (60%). It has also been suggested by Hemmings et al. that an element of *mandibular repo- sitioning involving the condyles* may also be occurring concomitantly.[28] Other phrases used to describe this concept include *minor axial tooth movement, fixed orthodontic intrusion, localised inter-occlusal space creation*, and *relative axial tooth movement*. The same principle may be extended to the controlled move- ment of posterior teeth to create space.[27]

According to a review by Poyser et al., when considering the studies that have assessed the efficacy of the Dahl concept, *a success rate of between 94 and 100% has been reported.*[27] Furthermore, the level of space creation appears to be con- sistent, irrespective of age and sex.[27] However, it would appear that careful *case selection with the placement of restorations in the supra-occlusal position is of paramount importance* when aiming for a successful outcome with the application of this concept.

Hemmings et al. have reported failures to also occur in patients with gross Class III malocclusions, with mandibular facial asymmetry, with a lack of stable occlusal contacts in either centric occlusion or CR.[28] The *lack of eruptive potential* should also be given due consideration. Patients who may display reduced eruptive potential (and may not be suitable for this form of intervention) include those presenting with:

- bony ankylosis
- dental implant restorations
- conventional fixed–fixed bridgework
- anterior open bites.

The application of the Dahl concept should also be undertaken with great caution amongst patients who may have/had:

- active/a past history of periodontal disease
- temporomandibular joint pain dysfunction syndrome
- endodontically teeth
- post-orthodontic treatment (as stability may become compromised).

Whilst there is little evidence in literature to suggest that the process of controlled intrusion and extrusion is associated with possible adverse effects such as pulpal symptoms, periodontal problems, TMJ dysfunction symptoms, and apical root resorption,[27] the feature of compliance with removable appliances has been identified as a true concern.[26]

To overcome the issues related to patient compliance (and aesthetic concerns of the removable prosthesis with visible clasp display), Ibbetson and Setchell[29] described an alternative approach involving the provision of a fixed metal prosthesis that is cemented in supra-occlusion with the same occlusal prescription as with the removable appliance with a glass ionomer lute or dual affinity cement. With the subsequent establishment of inter-occlusal clearance, the objective of the treatment plan was to replace the casting with conventional indirect castings.

The removal of the metallic backings may, however, occur at a risk of further compromising an already brittle, worn tooth. Furthermore, the preparation of such teeth to receive conventional restorations may have a negative impact on the pulpal status and the quantity of the remaining dental hard tissue.

As material technology has continued to evolve, it has now become acceptable to use tooth-coloured materials such as resin composite on the affected surfaces as a substitute for adhesively retained metal backings. Such composite restorations may be considered to be medium-term restorations (particularly where the wear is largely from erosive causes), and may offer a suitable means of restoring (especially the worn anterior dentition) by minimal intervention, concomitantly offering a satisfactory aesthetic outcome with the scope of contingency planning. Indeed, there is some good evidence to support the placement of restorations in a supra-occlusal position to help with the management of the worn dentition in a predictable manner concomitantly offering biological conservation (Figure 5.8). This evidence, together with the technical stages involved with the adoption of this concept in clinical practice, is discussed further in Chapters 10 and 11.

It should be noted, however, that when using the above concept, by definition, as the ICP will now be altered the process of placing a restoration in supra-occlusion would not involve the implementation of a conformative approach towards occlusal rehabilitation. However, whether in fact a *purist* approach towards the planning and making of restorations would ultimately aim for an ICP whereby the RCP and ICP would be reasonably co-incident (at the stage when the occlusal contacts have re-established) will depend on a number of factors, including:

- the pattern of wear present, whether affecting a single tooth, a small number of isolated teeth or indeed a large number of teeth (such as the anterior maxillary segment)
- the stability of the patient's ICP
- the actual discrepancy between ICP and RCP, and the broader implication of reorganising the occlusion.

In general, the operator should ultimately aim to place the restorations in a manner which gives due consideration to the requirements of the dental material being prescribed and the aesthetic and functional requirements of the patient (inclusive of comfort with mastication and phonation), and achieves a mechanically stable occlusal scheme as described in above.

5.7 Summary and Conclusions

In summary, it is important for the operator to have a good understanding of the essential theoretical and practical concepts in relation to clinical occlusion when embarking upon the restorative rehabilitation of a dentition displaying wear, especially when the pattern may involve the occluding surfaces. Whilst it may be argued that some of the concepts lack the support of evidence from the scientific literature, in general the consensus view is that they are based on a set of logical and well-accepted guidelines for good practice.[12] A gross departure from these guidelines may indeed form the basis of a standard of care that may be seen to have fallen far below a reasonable standard of expectation for a dental practitioner and may therefore prove indefensible in the event of a complaint being made.

As evidence is emerging for the success of the application of concepts that may represent a divergence from the traditional protocols, the ultimate goal remains to provide the patient with a stable occlusal scheme when undertaking restorative rehabilitation regardless of the approach taken.

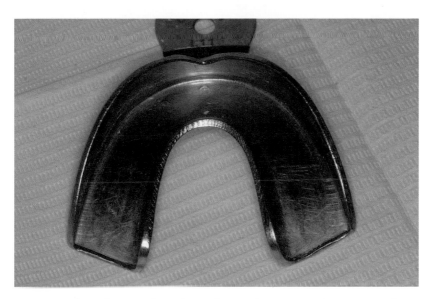

Figure 5.1 A rigid metal non-perforated rimlock tray. When using such a tray meticulous blocking out of undercuts present between the teeth and any hard tissues should be carried out to prevent locking of the tray following setting of the impression material.

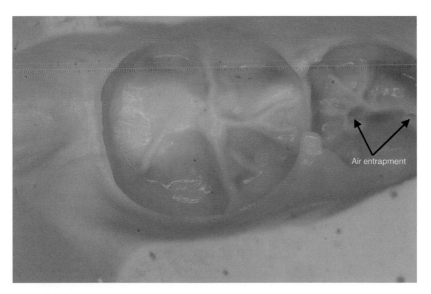

Figure 5.2 The impression should be carefully inspected for any defects. In this figure areas of air entrapment are highlighted.

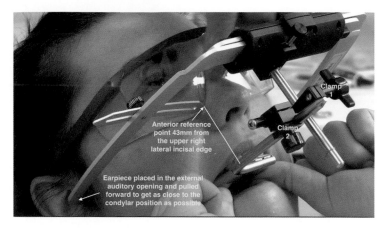

Figure 5.3 A facebow recording in position.

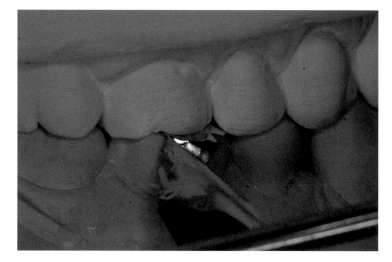

Figure 5.4 The contact between opposing teeth can be verified on the casts using articulating foil (Shimstock). These contacts, when in the same locations in the patient's dentition, will signify accuracy of the recordings and transfer.

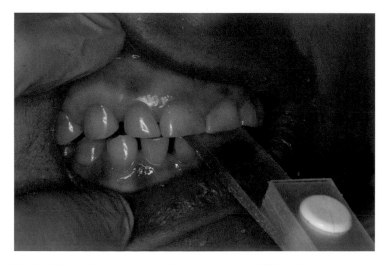

Figure 5.5 A Leaf Gauge in use to record the centric relation (CR) position.

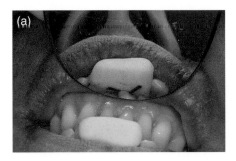
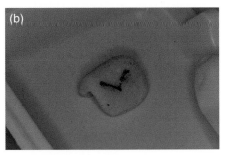

Figure 5.6 Use of a Lucia Jig. (a) The jig *in situ* in the patient and located on the upper incisor teeth. (b) The gothic arch tracing recorded. The apex of the tracing signifies the position of centric relation (CR).

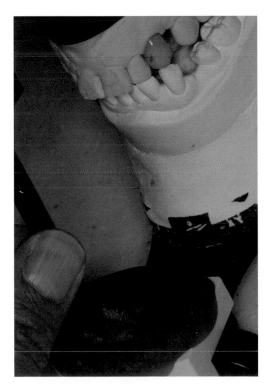

Figure 5.7 A customised incisal guidance table to help in the construction of an upper left canine crown.

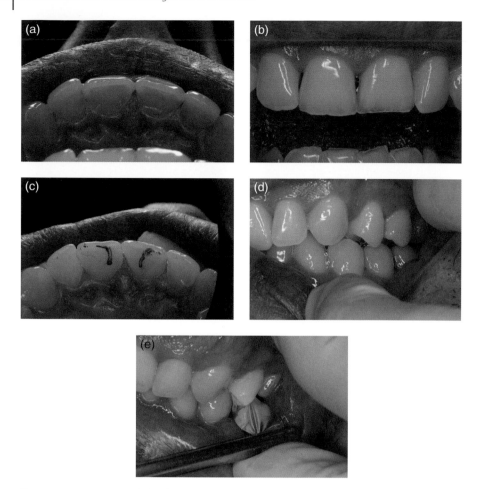

Figure 5.8 A patient with localised palatal incisal TW on the upper central incisors, which are sensitive and of an aesthetic concern to the patient. (a) Palatal view of the upper central incisors. (b) The labial view, note the incisal translucency. Direct composite has been added to the palatal surfaces of the upper central incisors without any tooth reduction and the protrusive guidance is distributed as depicted by the articulating paper markings in (c). (d) The posterior teeth are not in contact following the addition of the direct composite restorations on the upper central incisors. (e) Posterior contact has been re-established after a period of time and demonstrated by the posterior opposing teeth holding the articulating foil (Shimstock).

References

1 Davies, S. and Gray, R. (2001). What is occlusion? *Br. Dent. J.* 191: 235–245.
2 Davies, S., Gray, R., and Whitehead, S. (2001). Good practice in advanced restorative dentistry. *Br. Dent. J.* 191: 421–434.
3 Stuart, C. and Stallard, H. (1963). Concepts of occlusion. *Dent. Clin. N. Am.* 7: 591.
4 Milosevic, A. (2003). Occlusion: 2. Occlusal splints, analysis and adjustment. *Dent. Update* 30: 416–422.

5 Rosensteil, S., Land, M., and Fujimoto, J. (2006). *Contemporary Fixed Prosthodontics*, 4e. Mosby.

6 Beyron, H. (1969). Optimal occlusion. *Dent. Clin. N. Am.* 13: 537–554.

7 Eliyas, S. and Martin, N. (2013). The management of anterior tooth wear using gold palatal veneers in canine guidance. *Br. Dent. J.* 214: 291–297.

8 Koyano, K., Tsukiyama, Y., and Kuwatsuru, R. (2012). Rehabilitation of occlusion – science or art? *J. Oral Rehabil.* 39: 513–521.

9 Mehta, S.B., Banerji, S., Millar, B.J. et al. (2012). Current concepts on the management of tooth wear: Part 1. Assessment, treatment planning and strategies for the prevention and passive management of tooth wear. *Br. Dent. J.* 212: 17–27.

10 Patel, M. and Alani, A. (2015). Clinical issues in occlusion – Part II. *Singap. Dent. J.* 36: 2–11.

11 Milosevic, A. (2003). Occlusion 3: articulators and related instruments. *Dent. Update* 30: 511–515.

12 Davies, S. and Gray, R. (2001). The examination and recording of the occlusion: why and how. *Br. Dent. J.* 191: 291–302.

13 Whip Mix Corporation. The Denar Mark II System, Technique Manual. Whip Mix Corporation, Louisville, KY. www.whipmix.com.

14 Posselt, U. (1957). Movement areas of the mandible. *J. Prosthet. Dent.* 7 (3): 375–385.

15 Posselt, U. (1952). Studies in the mobility of the human mandible. *Acta Odotol. Scand.* 10 (Suppl 10).

16 Wilson, P. and Banerjee, A. (2004). Recording the retruded contact position: a review of the clinical techniques. *Br. Dent. J.* 196: 395–402.

17 Dawson, P.E. (1973). Temporomandibular joint pain dysfunction problems can be solved. *J. Prosthet. Dent.* 29: 100.

18 Wassell, R., Steele, J., and Welsh, G. (1998). Considerations when planning occlusal rehabilitation: a review of the literature. *Int. Dent. Jour.* 48: 571–581.

19 Berry, D. and Poole, D. (1976). Attrition: possible mechanisms of compensation. *J. Oral Rehabil.* 30: 201–206.

20 Loomans, B., Opdam, N., Attin, T. et al. (2017). Severe tooth wear: European consensus statement on management guidelines. *J. Adhes. Dent.* 19: 111–119.

21 Mehta, S.B., Banerji, S., Millar, B.J., and Saures-Fieto, J.M. (2012). Current concepts in tooth wear management. Part 3 active restorative care 2: the management of generalised tooth wear. *Br. Dent. J.* 212 (3): 121–127.

22 Celenza, F. (1973). The centric position: replacement and character. *J. Prosthet. Dent.* 30: 591–598.

23 Saunders, W. and Saunders, E. (1998). Prevalence of per-radicular periodontitis associated with crowned teeth in an adult Scottish subpopulation. *Br. Dent. J.* 185: 137–140.

24 Edlehoff, D. and Sorenssen, J. (2002). Tooth structure removal associated with various preparation designs for anterior teeth. *J. Prosthet. Dent.* 87: 503–509.

25 Dahl, B., Krungstad, O., and Karlsen, K. (1975). An alternative treatment of cases with advanced localised attrition. *J. Oral Rehabil.* 2: 209–214.

26 Dahl, B. and Krungstad, O. (1985). Long term observations of an increased occlusal face height obtained by a combined orthodontic/ prosthetic approach. *J. Oral Rehabil.* 12: 173–170.

27 Poyser, N., Porter, R., Briggs, P. et al. (2005). The Dahl concept: past, present and future. *Br. Dent. J.* 198: 669–676.

28 Hemmings, K., Darbar, U., and Vaughn, S. (2000). Tooth wear treated with direct composite at an increased vertical dimension: results at 30 months. *J. Prosthet. Dent.* 83: 287–293.

29 Ibbetson, R. and Setchell, D. (1989). Treatment of the worn dentition; 2. *Dent. Update* 16: 300–307.

Further Reading

Rosenstiel, S., Land, M., and Fujimoto, J. (2006). *Contemporary Fixed Prosthodontics*, 4e. Mosby.

Shillingburg, H., Sather, D., Wilson, E. et al. *Fundamentals of Fixed Prosthodontics*, 4e. Quintessence Publishing.

6

Management of Tooth Wear: Monitoring and Prevention Strategies

6.1 Introduction

Monitoring and prevention are important aspects to consider in the effective management of tooth wear (TW). Regardless of which operative procedure or intention is decided or indicated according to the patient's requirements, an effective prevention strategy to limit the further loss of tooth tissue along with careful monitoring of any progress is considered mandatory by the authors.

6.2 Counselling and Monitoring

If the amount of wear is physiological (typical for the age of the patient), no treatment will be needed. If the wear is pathological[1] further diagnostics are needed to determine the best management of it. Regardless of whether the TW can be defined as pathological or severe, people may be functioning with their worn dentition to their satisfaction for years. The advice to start an often complex rehabilitation treatment protocol for patients who have no functional problems or complaints may not be indicated, but careful monitoring of their dentition would be required. Patients with severe and pathological TW can be without actual complaints and therefore with further progression the restorative treatment may become compromised due to lack of retentive tooth tissue for adhesive restorations. Hence the first option for this group of patients is to start an effective monitoring and awareness strategy. This is preferred for cases where dentin is exposed and indices indicate the worst stages of wear. The reasons why monitoring is important include the following:

1) Patients with severe and pathological TW who do not perceive a need for any treatment and have no functional or aesthetic complaints are in a high-risk category for future restorative intervention due to the potential for continued tooth tissue loss. The adhesive potential for the remaining tooth tissue will become compromised and therefore may lead to failure of the restorations. Monitoring this process is invaluable for the clinician to anticipate this issue.

2) Effective monitoring is invaluable for patient awareness of the problem of their TW. Moderate to severe TW is not a linear process but manifests as

Practical Procedures in the Management of Tooth Wear, First Edition. Subir Banerji, Shamir Mehta, Niek Opdam and Bas Loomans.
© 2020 John Wiley & Sons Ltd. Published 2020 by John Wiley & Sons Ltd.
Companion website: www.wiley.com/go/banerji/toothwear

episodic, so monitoring the situation in a controllable way will lead to either the finding that wear is limited in progression and further monitoring is all that is required, or, when a clear progression of wear is demonstrated, the advice to start rehabilitation can be given with the likelihood of better patient compliance and understanding.

3) The monitoring process will also help the clinician to time the restorative treatment appropriately to slow down the restorative cycle process and contribute to a better lifelong management strategy for the worn dentition.

In patients who require restorative intervention, a minimally invasive adhesive approach should be considered as the first choice of treatment. Partial rehabilitation utilising the principles of passive axial tooth eruption (Dahl)[2] should be considered. This approach has been introduced as a concept in Chapter 5 and will be elaborated in subsequent ones. Further monitoring of the restored dentition is also desirable.

Counselling and monitoring are advised for the patients with severe or pathological wear. Counselling includes giving information to the patient about their TW and establishes an individual preventive programme, whereas monitoring includes the objective measurement of the amount of wear and its progression over time. Counselling and monitoring are much more than just assessing the amount of TW and involve certain important aspects:

1) A personalised identification of risk factors, mainly related to chemical or mechanical aetiology, should be done and explained to patients. Personalised preventive measures related to the patient's risk profile should be prescribed.

2) Analyses of wear progression. Teeth are designed to wear over a lifetime. However, TW is an episodic process consisting of inactive periods of physiological wear and active periods of progressive wear due to etiological factors like lifestyle, stomach acid, and bruxism.[3–5]

3) Patients should be aware that their wear is a personal problem related to their specific risk factors. The continued presence of these risk factors, when not dealt with preventively, will lead to future wear and possible deterioration of tooth tissue as well as any applied restorations. In addition, restorative treatment in, for example, severe bruxism cases will have a higher risk for fracturing restorations in case of rehabilitation. It is important that patients are aware of this risk before starting any restorative treatment: before treatment it is 'information', afterwards it is an 'excuse'.

4) Depending on the aetiology, amount, and progression of wear, and the feasibility of intended preventive measurements, a realistic expectation towards further monitoring or restorative treatments should be given to the patient.

To avoid a situation of supervised neglect it is most important that monitoring be accomplished according to specific protocols:

1) Diagnosis of the TW, including risk assessment related to the amount and aetiology of wear, should be noted in the patient file. The severity of TW can

be determined by using an index score, e.g. the Tooth Wear Index (TWI), the Basic Erosive Wear Examination (BEWE) or the Tooth Wear Evaluation System (TWES).[6–8]

2) The shared decision-making outcomes and the actions taken have to be added to the clinical records of the patient.

3) Monitoring can be performed by making a series of traditional casts (Figure 6.1) or digital 3D datasets/scans (Figure 6.2) of teeth obtained over a period of several months or years. These casts or digital 3D datasets are also a valuable aid to elucidate the aetiology of the process and explain the nature and severity of the condition to the patient and therefore increase the patient's awareness of the problem.

4) Depending upon the progression and severity of wear and the presence of functional or esthetical problems, new registrations can be made at intervals of approximately two to three years.[9] A schedule for re-evaluation should be noted In the patient's file.

If monitoring reveals that the wear process is progressive, this should signal the need for preventive measures or a referral for investigation of, for example, gastric reflux disease. It may also help reinforce patient acceptance of the need for compliance with an agreed care plan to preserve and, where indicated clinically, repair or possibly restore the damaged teeth. Engaging the patient in their monitoring protocol will lead to increased awareness of their problem, and also provide more insight into the severity and progression of the TW, leading to better future decisions on restorative treatments. All relevant decision making should be made in partnership with the patient. Factors such as pain or discomfort, and functional or aesthetic problems may, individually or collectively, be reason to embark on a programme of restorative care. When no demands, concerns or symptoms are present, a targeted preventative approach may be all that is required. In such cases, arrangements should be made for further counselling and monitoring. In the event of a patient having clinically insignificant amounts of wear for their age, and being found to be free of any active wear, the clinician should resist any request for restorative intervention from the patient. In all cases, the benefits of care must clearly outweigh any immediate or subsequent negative consequences. Above all else, patients must not be launched into an unnecessary 'restorative death spiral'[10] driven by failing restorations of ever-increasing complexity and cost.

In cases where the TW has progressed such that retention of possible restorations becomes a risk, for example when the crown height is reduced by more than two-thirds, the authors advise that the patient should be made well aware of the advantages of a rehabilitative approach even if the patient has no functional or aesthetic demands. However, it should be appreciated that a predictable and successful restorative intervention is always dependant on full commitment and valid informed consent. It needs to be considered that patients with extreme levels of TW may have a higher risk for restoration failure due to certain destructive parafunctional habits.

6.3   Prevention

Risk assessment is an important aspect of evidenced-based, patient-centred decision making in modern healthcare provision. Patients with severe TW should be risk assessed for possible alternative forms of management. Due consideration must be given to the effects of further wear and the failure of restorations and prostheses. In this respect, it is important to assess the likelihood of further wear and what form this wear may take. Episodes of wear may well have different aetiologies and rates of progression. As mechanical wear causing attrition or abrasion is enhanced by the initial demineralisation (softening) of dental hard tissue, TW is often described as erosive and involves both mechanical and chemical factors.

When aetiological factors are clear, like known gastro-oesophageal reflux disease (GORD), a diagnosis is established and a personalised preventive treatment can be administered.[11] However, in many cases of TW with the presence of signs of both mechanical or chemical factors, the specific aetiology cannot often be established. This makes the prognosis of TW as well as that of the possible restorative treatments unpredictable.

6.4   Preventive Measures in Case of Chemical Wear

Counselling starts with identifying the risk factors. A nightguard should be considered in cases where clenching and grinding are contributory. Dietary advice, discussing drinking and eating habits, or referring the patient to a gastroenterologist in case of a suspicion for GORD will need to be considered. Dietary advice may include reducing the amount and frequency of intake of acidic drinks, changing drinking habits (such as 'swishing' or 'sipping'), using drinking straws, and advising safer food alternatives, such as calcium-enriched (sports) drinks and foods, and drinking non-carbonated water and milk.[12]

In case of erosive aetiology, it is possible to use specific protective products or materials, such as toothpastes or mouth rinses containing stannous fluoride or stannous chloride, which have the potential for slowing the progression of erosive TW.[13] However, there is limited evidence for the efficacy of the long-term use of toothpastes or changing dietary habits.

In cases where gastric acid is established as the aetiological factor, for example in GORD patients, preventive measures follow guidelines for reflux patients, such as losing weight, a low-fat diet, avoiding spicy foods, adjusting the sleeping position by raising the head during sleep etc. For patients diagnosed with GORD, proton-pump inhibitors may be prescribed which may have a preventive effect and will slow down further TW.[14] However, currently there is no evidence available indicating the reduction of TW whilst using proton pomp inhibitors (PPI) over a longer period of time. As often severe

TW patients suffer from multifactorial aetiological factors, preventive measures can be increasingly complex as gastric acid may have a worsening effect when retained inside a nightguard during the night. Therefore, in severe TW cases the prognosis of the treatment and the effect of specific preventive measures is often difficult to determine as diagnosis are often 'best guesses' and evidence for preventive measures is inadequate.

6.5   Preventive Measures in Case of Mechanical Wear

In those patients diagnosed with severe bruxing habits as the main etiological factor for TW, prevention is important for both the natural dentition as well as the restorative material. First, patients should be made aware of their bruxing habits. Self-reported bruxism may not be a reliable indicator as patients may consider this daily routine as 'normal'. Therefore it is important to explain to patients that opposing teeth should only make contact during swallowing, and this may make the patient more aware of a bruxing habit. Myo-feedback therapy has been shown to play a role in the prevention of awake bruxism. Patient must be made aware that persistent bruxism, both during sleeping and whilst awake,[15] may also limit the prognosis of restorations fabricated from inherently brittle materials, for example ceramic onlays and crowns.

A nightguard may be valuable to be used to protect tooth structures and restorations, although the prevention of either further TW or damage to restorations has never been proven in clinical studies. The disadvantage of a nightguard is the need for a compliant patient, and therefore patients should be informed about the possible discomfort and the need to get accustomed to the device. After restorative rehabilitation in an increased vertical dimension, a further increased bite due to the nightguard may enhance the perception of discomfort and this should be communicated to the patient. The designs of these devices are discussed in Chapter 7.

Many cases of severe TW are multifactorial in their origin, which makes the prescription of adequate prevention regimes difficult and challenging. Often the multi-factorial origin of severe TW prevents a clear diagnosis of the etiological factors. Moreover, taking away all the aetiological factors by a prevention regime may be unrealistic when dealing with patients suffering from, for example, long-established, recalcitrant chronic reflux disease[16] or persistent bruxism.[17]

In cases where the aetiological factors are unclear and preventive measures are not much more than a best guess, these measures should be continually reviewed to avoid precipitating any further harm. Nightguards have the potential for increased erosive TW in patients with nocturnal reflux, and the side effects of proton-pump inhibitors, even in established cases of reflux, are a serious consideration when embarking on a lifelong preventive therapy regime.[18]

Figure 6.3 shows the flow of the steps involved in the management of TW.

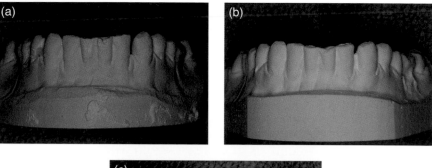

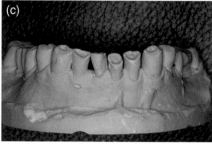

Figure 6.1 Stone study casts to monitor the TW in the lower dentition of a patient: (a) September 2003, (b) May 2007, and (c) July 2012. Notice the marked TW on the lower anterior incisor teeth between May 2007 and July 2012.

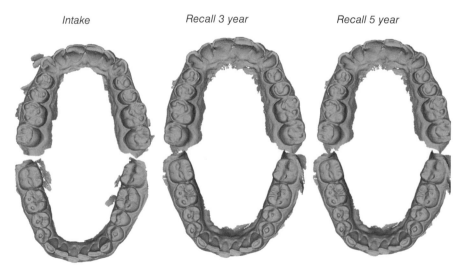

Figure 6.2 Digital scans to monitor the progression of TW. Male, 44 years old. After 5 years, progression of TW led to functional problems and restorative treatment was started.

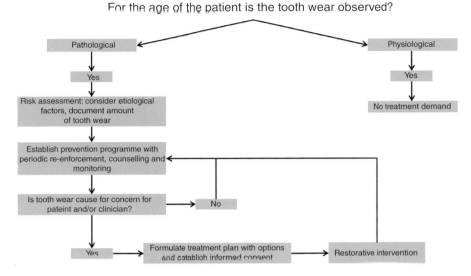

Figure 6.3 Flowchart showing an overview of the management of TW.

References

1 Loomans, B., Opdam, N., Attin, T. et al. (2017). Severe Tooth Wear: European Consensus Statement on Management Guidelines. *J. Adhes. Dent.* 19: 111–119.

2 Dahl, B.L., Krogstad, O., and Karlsen, K. (1975). An alternative treatment of cases with advanced localized attrition. *J. Oral Rehabil.* 2: 209–214.

3 Bartlett, D. (2008). Pathological or physiological erosion – is there a relationship to age? *Clin. Oral Investig.* 12 (suppl 1): S27–S31.

4 Kisely, S., Sawyer, E., Siskind, D., and Lallo, R. (2016). The oral health of people with anxiety and depressive disorders – a systematic review and meta-analysis. *J. Affect. Disord.* 200: 119–132.

5 Ahmed, K.E. (2013). The psychology of tooth wear. *Spec. Care Dentist.* 33: 28–34. Review.

6 Smith, B.G.N. and Knight, J.K. (1984). An index for measuring the wear of teeth. *Br. Dent. J.* 156: 435–438.

7 Bartlett, D., Ganss, C., and Lussi, A. (2008). Basic Erosive Wear Examination (BEWE): a new scoring system for scientific and clinical needs. *Clin. Oral Investig.* 12 (Suppl 1): S65–S68.

8 Wetselaar, P. and Lobbezoo, F. (2016). The tooth wear evaluation system: a modular clinical guideline for the diagnosis and management planning of worn dentitions. *J. Oral Rehabil.* 43: 69–80.

9 Loomans, B. and Opdam, N. (2018 Mar 9). A guide to managing tooth wear: the Radboud philosophy. *Br. Dent. J.* 224 (5): 348–356.

10 Elderton, R.J. (1990). Clinical studies concerning re-restoration of teeth. *Adv. Dent. Res.* 4 (1): 4–9.

11 Moazzez, R. and Bartlett, D. (2014). Intrinsic causes of erosion. *Monogr. Oral Sci.* 25: 180–196.

12 Carvalho, T.S., Lussi, A., Jaeggi, T., and Gambon, D.L. (2014). Erosive tooth wear in children. *Monogr. Oral Sci.* 25: 262–278.

13 West, N.X., He, T., Macdonald, E.L. et al. (2017). Erosion protection benefits of stabilized SnF2 dentifrice versus an arginine-sodium monofluorophosphate dentifrice: results from in vitro and in situ clinical studies. *Clin. Oral Investig.* 21: 533–540.

14 Wilder-Smith, C.H., Wilder-Smith, P., Kawakami-Wong, H. et al. (2009 Nov). Quantification of dental erosions in patients with GERD using optical coherence tomography before and after double-blind, randomized treatment with esomeprazole or placebo. *Am. J. Gastroenterol.* 104 (11): 2788–2795.

15 Lobbezoo, F., Ahlberg, J., Raphael, K.G. et al. (2018). International consensus on the assessment of bruxism: Report of a work in progress. *J. Oral Rehabil.* 45 (11): 837–844.

16 Wilder-Smith, C.H., Materna, A., Martig, L., and Lussi, A. (2015). Gastro-oesophageal reflux is common in oligosymptomatic patients with dental erosion: A pH-impedance and endoscopic study. *United European Gastroenterol J* 3: 174–181.

17 Van de Sande, F.H., Collares, K., Correa, M.B. et al. (2016). Restoration survival: revisiting patients' risk factors through a systematic literature review. *Oper. Dent.* 41 (suppl 7): S7–S26.

18 Corleto, V.D., Festa, S., Di Giulio, E., and Annibale, B. (2014 Feb). Proton pump inhibitor therapy and potential long-term harm. *Curr. Opin. Endocrinol. Diabetes Obes.* 21 (1): 3–8.

7

The Role of Occlusal Splints for Patients with Tooth Wear

7.1 Introduction

Occlusal splints (also referred to as occlusal devices) may be defined as 'any removable artificial occlusal surface affecting the relationship of the mandible to the maxillae used for diagnosis or therapy'.[1]

There is a large array of such appliances that serve a variety of different purposes in clinical dentistry. For descriptive purposes, they may be classified according to their *level of coverage* (full versus partial), their *consistency* (hard or soft), the *arch* to which they may be applied or whether they *reposition the mandible* into a pre-determined position or are flat, thus of the *stabilisation variety*.

This chapter focuses on the role of stabilisation splints for the management of tooth wear (TW), but the use of soft, full coverage occlusal splints will also be discussed.

7.2 The Role of Stabilisation Splints for the Management of Tooth Wear

A stabilisation splint essentially provides the patient with a removable ideal occlusal scheme according to the principals of the *mutually protected occlusal scheme*, as discussed in Chapter 5. Such devices should provide:[2]

- even contact with all the antagonistic teeth in the arc of closure when the mandibular condyles are physiologically seated in the glenoid fossae
- a lighter level of contact with the anterior dentition than with the posterior teeth
- smooth and ready separation (disclusion) of the posterior teeth on occlusal contact being formed between the anterior teeth and the occlusal device upon lateral and protrusive mandibular movement.

To permit the above, and to also allow for even force distribution across the dental arches as well as to prevent unwanted over-eruption of antagonistic teeth, the stabilisation splint must offer a *complete/full-arch design*.[3]

Practical Procedures in the Management of Tooth Wear, First Edition. Subir Banerji, Shamir Mehta, Niek Opdam and Bas Loomans.
© 2020 John Wiley & Sons Ltd. Published 2020 by John Wiley & Sons Ltd.
Companion website: www.wiley.com/go/banerji/toothwear

The maxillary stabilisation splint is commonly referred to as a *Michigan splint* (Figures 7.1–7.6) whilst the mandibular stabilisation splint is often termed a *Tanner appliance* (Figures 7.7 and 7.8). Whilst both offer an analogous outcome, the latter are perhaps more suitable for patients displaying a Class III incisor relationship (as it may prove easier to develop the desired occlusal scheme) or where the tolerance of a maxillary appliance may be of concern.

The prescription of a stabilisation occlusal splint for the worn dentition may be considered:

- for the protection of the natural and/or restored dentition during parafunctional (bruxist) activity
- for the management of myogenous orofacial pain[4]
- for the diagnosis of occlusal pathology
- for the stabilisation of the occlusal scheme prior to complex restorative care provision, including the assessment of patient tolerance to an occlusal scheme, with an altered vertical occlusal dimension
- when attempting to providing passive (preventative) management for cases of pathological TW where attrition due to bruxism is a likely significant cause[5]
- when attempting to locate (and/or reposition a patient into) centric relation
- as part of the process of attempting to create inter-occlusal clearance by relative axial tooth movement (occlusal adaptation) for cases such as those displaying TW.

The ability to prescribe and construct a stabilisation splint has therefore many potential merits for the restorative dentist.

The precise method(s) by which a stabilisation splint can fulfil some of its established merits is/are unknown. However, it has been suggested that the effect of posterior disclusion (as offered by a stabilisation splint) results in a decrease in elevator muscle hyperactivity.[6] Furthermore, electromyographic studies have described a reduction in anterior temporalis and master muscle activity when clenching on a canine ramp, as opposed to when performing the same role during group function or centric occlusal contact.[6,7] As discussed below, the inclusion of a canine ramp is one of the key design features of such appliances.

To permit the fabrication of an occlusal device that offers the above function, traditional techniques have relied on the use of resilient materials such as a *heat-cured polymethyl methacrylate (PMMA)*, often of a transparent variety. This can culminate in a durable appliance, which may be suitably contoured to the desired prescription, readily adjusted, and will be minimally abrasive towards antagonistic surfaces.

However, with the increasing popularity of CAD/CAM in dentistry, it is also possible to use alternative more flexible tooth-coloured, polycarbonate-based materials to provide occlusal appliances, which offer acceptable levels of fracture resistance at comparatively lower levels of thickness and may prove invaluable amongst patients where compliance and tolerance with bulkier appliances may be problematic.[8] These will also be briefly overviewed as part of this chapter.

7.3   Clinical Protocol for the Fabrication of a Stabilisation Splint: The Conventional Approach

The account provided below relates to the construction of a *Michigan splint*, but the same concepts can be applied to a mandibular stabilisation splint.

Accurate impressions and occlusal records are imperative to the provision of an accurate and well-fitting occlusal device. Whilst the use of custom trays with appropriate impression materials is ideal, the use of metal rim lock impression trays with an accurate alginate-based impression material may prove more time- and cost-effective, provided that the impressions are cast relatively quickly and in a suitable, dimensionally stable material. Alginate is usually sufficient for the opposing arch, but an addition-cured polyviloxane silicone (PVS) is ideal for the working model. The use of a PVS material enables a duplicate cast to be poured to check the fit of the finished splint as the working cast is often damaged during splint construction.

Prior to the taking of the impression, it is important to ensure that the occlusal surfaces are clean and suitably dried. Following the attainment of the impression, the latter should be closely inspected and excessive material at the borders carefully trimmed away.

Once the impressions have been cast, the casts should be permitted to dry for 24 hours after pouring prior to the undertaking of any anatomical articulation to provide the desired level of abrasion resistance.

The clinical techniques for the taking of a facebow record and an inter-occlusal record (to permit mounting on a semi-adjustable articulator) were alluded to in Chapter 5. Such occlusal records together with a clear and comprehensive laboratory prescription relating to the design of the appliance are fundamental to success.

In relation to the appliance thickness, splints formed from PMMA are usually fabricated to provide a minimal thickness (inter-occlusal clearance) of 1.5–2.0 mm. In the event of a patient displaying pathological TW, the thickness of the appliance may be dictated by the space requirements proposed for the rehabilitation.

To facilitate manufacture, an outline of the splint should be scribed onto the maxillary cast, ideally to extend approximately 3–4 mm onto the palate, 3 mm onto the buccal cusps of the posterior teeth, and with 2 mm of overlap of the incisal edges of the anterior teeth. Whilst gross undercut areas may need to be appropriately blocked out, the unnecessary blocking out of all undercuts on the proximal, buccal, and palatal surfaces should be avoided as the engagement of the acrylic-based materials into these interstitial areas will provide the necessary mechanical retention to retain the splint *in situ*. Where retention form may be a concern the addition of Adam cribs to engage the first molar teeth can be considered.

Sheets of softened pink baseplate wax should then be adapted to an adequately dampened maxillary cast to conform to the outline described above. The articulator is closed such that the incisal pin is in contact with the incisal table; this contact is verified by a positive tugging action on a piece of thin 8 μm articulating foil interposed between the pin and table. This will result in indentations into the wax base, thereby forming the centric stops. Excess wax is then cut away. The occluding surface should be relatively flat so that there is no potential for the cusps of the opposing dentition to be locked and they are able to move freely across the splint's occluding surface. A minimum of one centric stop should be present per opposing tooth. This may be verified using articulating paper.

Wax is then carefully added in the canine areas, positioned anterior to the established centric stops (to avoid an unwanted alteration in the occlusal prescription established so far) at an approximate angle of 45° to the occlusal surface. The *canine rise* formed should provide guidance to the mandible upon protrusive and excursive movements, ensuring separation of all other teeth. The canine risers are then connected by the further addition of wax in the anterior segment to form a shallow concave ramp that should provide immediate disclusion of the posterior teeth upon mandibular protrusion, with anterior guidance being shared equally between the anterior teeth.

At this stage, some clinicians elect to carry out a wax try-in. However, most often the wax pattern is processed and finished using a transparent heat-cured acrylic. It is also advisable to use a duplicate cast for processing to enable the splint to be repositioned onto the mounted casts for verification and final adjustments.

On receipt from the laboratory, the stabilisation splint should be carefully inspected and if deemed satisfactory, it should be inserted onto the patient's maxillary arch. If the splint is tight, such areas should be carefully relieved using an acrylic trimming bur. The use of an occlusal indicator medium such as Occlude Aerosol Indicator Marking Spray (Pascal Co. Inc.) to identify any areas of interference can prove particularly helpful in some cases.

Under circumstances where it has become possible to seat the splint with the appliance concomitantly displaying signs of minor instability, the option may be taken to reline the splint in this area using an appropriate chairside, cold-cured acrylic reline material.

Once the splint has been seated, and deemed to be adequately retentive, the use of a suitable form of articulating paper such as GHM Occlusion foil 12 μm (Hanel, Coltene Whaledent, Germany) is often advocated for marking up the centric stops. A higher level of accuracy may be offered by the use of computerised occlusal analysis (Tscan 3, Tekscan, Boston, USA). However, given that most clinicians in general dental practice/primary care settings will not have digital occlusal analysis apparatus at their disposal, the use of articulating paper/foil is deemed reasonable. Accordingly, for a right-handed operator, the articulating paper should be supported using a pair of Millers forceps in the left hand, and the patient requested to 'close together'. With the right hand positioned on the patient's chin, the clinician should gently guide the mandible into position along its retruded arc of closure. With the opposing teeth contacting the splint, the patient should be asked to rub slightly back and forth onto the splint in partial protrusive and excursive movements of the mandible.

The splint should then be removed from the patient's mouth. Using a sharp pencil, any desired areas of contact should be marked up; ideally, a minimum of one contact should exist between opposing functional cusps. Using an acrylic trimming bur or a wheel, any unwanted occlusal contacts should be carefully removed, whilst avoiding the creation of any unwanted indentations into the occluding surface. The splint should also be regularly checked (using an Ivanson's calliper) to ensure that it does not reach any less than a minimal thickness of 0.5 mm in any area, which will be necessary to make sure that it remains sufficiently robust to withstand occlusal loading.

Where an obvious lack of occlusal contact exists, there will be a need to add suitable increments of cold-cured acrylic onto the occluding surface of the splint, making sure that the patient is carefully manipulated into position and the established vertical dimension maintained.

Once the presence of centric stops has been identified between each occluding pair using articulating paper, these should be reassessed using an 8 µm articulating foil. Contacts should be lighter between opposing anterior teeth.

Next (using a different colour of articulating paper for visual clarity), the presence of a suitable canine rise that permits posterior disclusion on protrusion and lateral excursive movements should be ascertained (and confirmed). If inadequate, cold-cured resin may need to be added. However, the presence of a very steep rise should be duly avoided, as this may be poorly tolerated by the patient.

Finally, using a third colour of articulating paper it is imperative to establish the presence of evenly shared anterior guidance on protrusion and amend the splint accordingly, if initially deemed suboptimal.

In cases where the appliance is being provided to evaluate tolerance to a new occlusal scheme, the patient should be instructed to wear the appliance continually (other than when eating) for a period of one to three months. For cases where it has been prescribed for the control of nocturnal bruxism, the patient should be instructed to wear the splint every night until the recall appointment.

Patients should be reviewed after two weeks. The comfort, compliance to wear, and occlusal contacts should be verified at this appointment. It is likely that at this visit a discrepancy may be noted due to mandibular repositioning, as muscle relaxation may be taking place. A further review is recommended after a period of two weeks and adjustments made to the occlusal form until the stage where occlusal contacts are consistent between consecutive visits and the patient is comfortable.

7.4   The Use of CAD/CAM for Fabrication of a Stabilisation Splint

According to Edelhoff et al.[8] at the laboratory level, the use of 3D CAD/CAM technology to form a resilient occlusal splint (using traditional as well as more contemporary materials) can offer several advantages:

- the avoidance of polymerisation shrinkage (and its effect on the accuracy of the definitive appliance), which occurs when curing PMMA
- the scope to use prefabricated materials that have been optimally fabricated to industrial standards
- the potential to form a new appliance/second device on a master record, a process that may not be possible using conventional techniques when the

working casts may have sustained damage during the construction of the appliance (without the need to take new patient records).

In relation to the use of *tooth-coloured CAD/CAM polycarbonate*, in addition to some of the merits listed in the Introduction as well as the obvious aesthetic gains, given that stabilisation appliances fabricated using this material can be made to a minimum thickness of 0.3 mm, the option for the fitting of *two opposing splints* to further simulate the occlusal contours of a wax-up becomes possible (amongst cases where significant changes in the occlusal vertical dimension (OVD) are being planned, where an increase in the height of the incisal pin by 4 mm or more is required).[8] The use of separate splints in this manner can also permit a *segment-by segment* approach, allowing each arch to be treated separately/in a staged manner, with the presence of a splint at the unprepared arch permitting the continual existence of a mutually protective occlusal scheme.

The technique for the fabrication of a *removable polycarbonate splint* for a case requiring an increase in the OVD has been described by Edelhoff et al.[8] In summary, the protocol entails the following:

- The preparation of an appropriate diagnostic wax-up, followed by an intra-oral mock up (as detailed in Chapter 8).
- The scanning of the baseline casts and duplicate casts of the wax-up, followed by the positing of the models into a virtual articulator.
- Determination of the (cervical) length of the splint using the diagnostic model and the path of insertion/the presence of undercuts.
- The use of the wax-up to ascertain the static and dynamic occlusal form of the appliance, using the virtual articulator to correct any premature contacts that may have been introduced during the process of forming the wax-up.
- Use of CAM for the milling of the appliance.
- Finishing and polishing stages to achieve a high lustre.
- Try-in/fitting (as described above), to also include phonetic testing.

This approach has some advantages, but the financial cost of care may prove prohibitive.

7.5 The Use of Soft (Vacuum-formed) Occlusal Splints for the Management of TW

Soft splints are vacuum/thermoformed from ethylene-vinyl acetate (EVA).[9] Whilst they offer the merits of lower financial cost and ease of fabrication when compared with a hard, full coverage stabilisation appliance, there are several disadvantages associated with them, including:

- a tendency to wear down/perforate (especially amongst those displaying severe bruxist tendencies)
- a tendency to discolour with time
- difficult to adjust

- do not provide a specific occlusal scheme, with the concomitant risk of unwanted tooth movement
- scope to exacerbate muscle activity due to the presence of premature tooth contacts.[10]

Consequently, such splints are perhaps best used for the short-term protection of teeth/restorations from the effects of bruxism.

More recently, the prescription of *hybrid/bilaminar splints* with a soft inner layer (to offer a more comfortable fit) and a harder outer layer to offer a higher level of resilience has gained popularity.[5] In the experience of the authors, some types can display the separation of the two layers in areas of higher loading (especially where the thickness may be reduced), but other types of bilaminar splints (e.g. Somnobrux), in which a softer layer in the inside is embedded in a hard PMMA-matrix, are very good. These are often thicker splints compared to conventional splints, but have a much better fitting, no clamps, and patient's commitment is much better than with hard splints.

7.6   Summary and Conclusion

Occlusal splints have a variety of roles for the management of patients with TW. It is important that the clinician is familiar with the indications and mode of construction of a stabilisation splint. The role of the latter will be considered further in Chapter 13 on the management of generalised TW.

The accompanying video will describe the construction of an upper full arch (Michigan) stabilisation splint and the points mentioned in this chapter (www.wiley.com/go/banerji/toothwear).

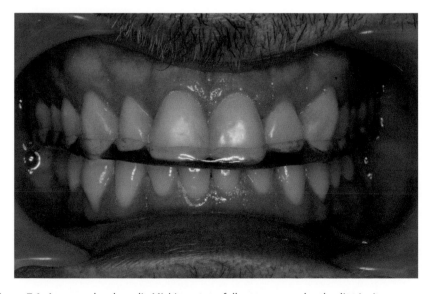

Figure 7.1   An upper hard acrylic Michigan-type full-coverage occlusal splint *in situ*.

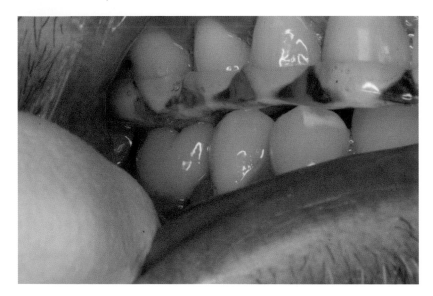

Figure 7.2 The splint in Figure 7.1 with the lower teeth in contact with the splint. Note the even contact of all the teeth and the lack of indentations in the splint where the lower teeth cusps are in contact with the splint surface.

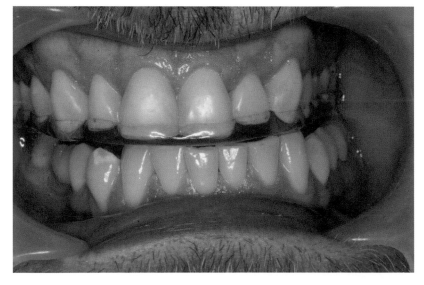

Figure 7.3 The patient from Figures 7.1 and 7.2 going into left excursion mandibular motion. Note disclusion of the posterior teeth.

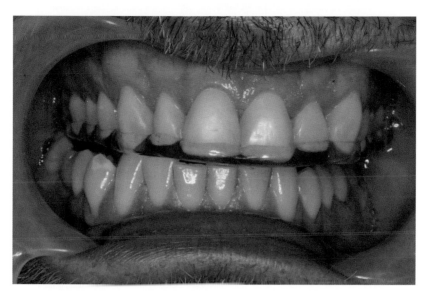

Figure 7.4 The patient from Figures 7.1 and 7.2 going into right excursion mandibular motion. Note disclusion of the posterior teeth.

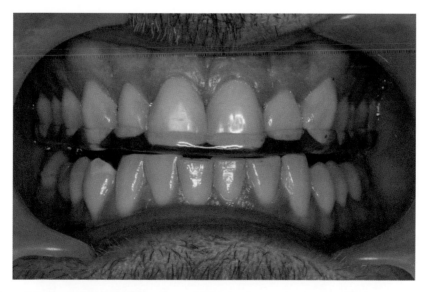

Figure 7.5 The patient from Figures 7.1 and 7.2 going into protrusive mandibular motion. Note disclusion of the posterior teeth.

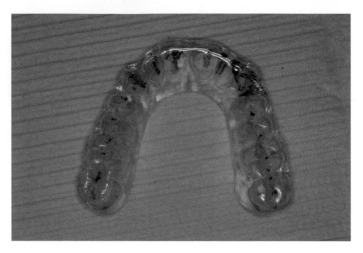

Figure 7.6 The occlusal contacts marked with articulating paper on the splint for the patient from Figure 7.1. Note the even centric contact marks with all the lower teeth and the excursive contacts on the anterior platform of the splint.

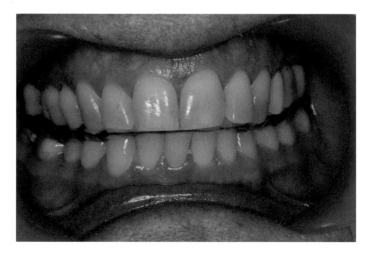

Figure 7.7 A lower hard acrylic Tanner-type full-coverage occlusal splint *in situ*.

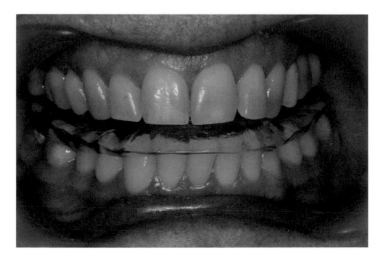

Figure 7.8 The patient from Figure 7.7 going into protrusive mandibular motion. Note disclusion of the posterior teeth.

References

1 The Academy of Prosthodontics Foundation (2017). The glossary of prosthodontic terms, 9th edition, GPT-9. *J. Prosthet. Dent.* 117 (5S): e1–e105.
2 Solow, R. (2013). Customized anterior guidance for occlusal devices: classification and rationale. *J. Prosthet. Dent.* 110: 259–263.
3 Milosevic, A. (2003). Occlusion: 2. Occlusal splints, analysis and adjustment. *Dent. Update* 30: 416–422.
4 Clark, G. (1984). A critical evaluation of orthopaedic interocclusal appliance therapy: design, theory and overall effectiveness. *J. Am. Dent. Assoc.* 108: 359–364.
5 Rees, J. and Somi, S. (2018). A guide to the clinical management of attrition. *Br. Dent. J.* 224: 319–323.
6 Manns, A., Chac, C., and Miralles, R. (1987). Influence of group function and canine guidance on electromyographic activity of elevator muscles. *J. Prosthet. Dent.* 57: 494–501.
7 Fitins, D. and Sheikoleslam, A. (1993). Effect of canine guidance of maxillary occlusal splint on level of activation of masticatory muscles. *Swed. Dent. J.* 17: 235–241.
8 Edelhoff, D., Schweiger, J., Prandtner, O. et al. (2017). CAD/CAM splints for the functional and esthetic evaluation of newly defined occlusal dimensions. *Quintessence Int.* 48: 181–191.
9 Green, J. (2016). Prevention and management of tooth wear. The role of dental technology. *Prim. Dent. J.* 5: 30–33.
10 Okeson, J. (1987). The effects of hard and soft occlusal splints on nocturnal bruxism. *J. Am. Dent. Assoc.* 114: 788–791.

Further Reading

Capp, N.J. Occlusion and splint therapy. In: *Tooth Surface Loss* (eds. R. Ibbetson and A. Eder) Chpt 3, 15–20. BDJ Books.

8

Treatment Planning and the Application of Diagnostic Techniques

8.1 Introduction

Having carried out the necessary diagnostic assessments and discussed all of the reasonable possible treatment options for a patient presenting with pathological tooth wear (TW), the clinician will be at a stage that will permit the development of an appropriately structured treatment plan. This should be based on the overarching aims of restoring the patient's oral health and function, as well as providing an acceptable aesthetic outcome. The process of treatment planning should give due consideration to the longer-term needs of that particular patient, and where possible be tailored to meet their bespoke needs.

A logically sequenced dental treatment plan should usually include a number of well-recognised stages.[1] These are listed in Table 8.1. It is incumbent on the treating clinician to periodically assess the efficacy of each stage of the treatment plan (prior to progressing to the next stage), as well as to ensure that the patient fully understands their overall responsibility towards the ultimate success of the prescribed plan, including the importance of longer-term maintenance and monitoring.

There are a number of factors that will influence the process of formulating a treatment plan for a patient with pathological TW, especially given the complex nature of treatment that may sometimes be required. These include:

- the standard of dentist–patient communication
- the patient's overall levels of motivation and their ability to understand the underlying issues and proposed treatment options
- the likely time frame required to complete the proposed course of care and the frequency of attendance
- the financial costs involved (which may be high, given that several teeth are often involved)[2]
- the level of operator skill/knowledge/confidence and experience.

The importance of the processes involved with the attainment of valid informed consent to treatment for a patient with TW cannot be overstated. It is also important that complete and contemporaneous clinical records are maintained throughout the delivery of patient care.

Practical Procedures in the Management of Tooth Wear, First Edition. Subir Banerji, Shamir Mehta, Niek Opdam and Bas Loomans.
© 2020 John Wiley & Sons Ltd. Published 2020 by John Wiley & Sons Ltd.
Companion website: www.wiley.com/go/banerji/toothwear

Table 8.1 The various stages of a well-structured dental treatment plan.[1]

1) Management of the acute complaint

2) Initiation of the preventative protocol

3) Disease control and stabilisation

4) Review of the preventative compliance and disease control status

5) Pre-rehabilitative assessment

6) Oral rehabilitation, including complex restorations

7) Maintenance, recall, and monitoring

The aims of this chapter are to:

- overview the activities that take place during each aspect of the execution of the treatment plan
- list the criteria where active restorative intervention is indicated amongst patients presenting with TW
- provide an account of the clinical stages required to fabricate the occlusal-aesthetic prescription, focusing on the preparation of a diagnostic wax-up (Figure 8.1). This is a helpful tool in helping to gain informed consent for the proposed treatment plan.

8.2 Developing a Logically Sequenced Treatment Plan for a Patient with Pathological Tooth Wear

For any patient presenting to the dental operatory with a diagnosis of pathological TW (as defined in Chapter 1), the primary aim should be the appropriate management of any acute conditions, hence the *emergency stage*. Treatment for the TW patient during this stage may include the simple application of a proprietary varnish to seal patent dentinal tubules, the placement of a dentine bonding agent or sealant restoration to help manage dentinal hypersensitivity and/or signs of reversible pulpitis, the prescription of chemical therapeutic agents, the placement of a composite bandage to treat a chipped/fractured tooth, the adjustment of a sharp surface that may be causing mucosal trauma, extirpation of an inflamed dental pulp, drainage of a swelling and the extraction of a symptomatic tooth.[3,4] The risks of dentinal hypersensitivity and endodontic complications amongst patients presenting with severe TW are addressed in Chapter 3.

It is generally accepted that active restorative intervention can only be successful beyond the short term where the patient and clinician have been collectively effective in preventing the aetiological factor from causing further deterioration of the patient's oral health. Preventative care should always be advised for patients with pathological TW regardless of the severity of the observed extent and pattern of wear seen.[5] Unfortunately, however, the importance attached to the *preventative phase* can sometimes be overlooked.

Preventative care prescription for patients with pathological wear should be tailored according to the underlying aetiology and symptoms, and may include diet advice, habit and lifestyle modification, oral hygiene instruction, fluoride application, the protection of surfaces with sealant type restorations, provision of an occlusal splint and referral to a medical practitioner where an underlying medical condition may be aetiological.[3] The topic of preventative care for the TW patient is discussed in depth in Chapter 6.

Having applied the appropriate forms of preventative care, it is vital to assess the efficacy of this phase. Specifically, in relation to the condition of TW such evaluations may include an appraisal of any habit changes, the cessation in the progression of the pattern of TW, the level of success with the management of any symptoms relating to pain and discomfort, the effective management of xerostomia, the taking of any required prescription medication/medical treatment, as well as an appraisal of the compliance with any prescribed dental treatment(s), such as occlusal splint therapy, The available means for monitoring the progression of TW in general include the use of casts, digital monitoring resources/intra-oral scanners, intra-oral photography and/or suitable clinical indexes. These are discussed in Chapters 4 and 6.

The period of time required to undertake an evaluation of the efficacy of the preventative phase is variable. It may range from a few weeks to several months depending on the nature and extent of the pathology (or aetiological factors) and the compliance of the patient. Preferably, definitive restorative treatment should not be provided until it has been established that the aetiological factors have been properly managed and the patient has displayed the required levels of compliance and success with the preventative regime.[6]

Indeed, active restorative intervention should be deferred for as long as reasonably possible. This measure will not only serve to delay the entry of the patient into the cycle of restorative care and maintenance, but also, given that TW is generally slowly progressive (thereby concomitantly alleviating the demands on the dental operator to commence immediate restorative treatment),[4] the time taken to ensure effective cessation of the TW pattern (prior to the commencement of active restorative intervention where indicated) may:

- allow enhancement of the dentist-patient relationship
- enable the patient to further understand the nature of their problem
- enable the complexities/challenges involved with restorative intervention of a severely worn dentition to be understood
- enhance the probability of achieving a long-term predictable outcome.

The exception to the above may be in the case of a younger dental patient, where the rate of TW (as seen in some cases of bulimia nervosa) may be very rapid, often associated with symptoms of sensitivity, the imminent risk of pulp tissue encroachment, as well as aesthetic compromise (due to the hasty loss of tooth tissue in the region of the aesthetic zone). The latter can have a profoundly deleterious impact on the longer-term state of patient oral health and general well-being, thus under such circumstances restorative treatment may need to be implemented without any further undue delay.[4,6]

The next phase of the treatment plan would normally involve the *stabilisation* of the effects of the pathology. This may also entail the management of other forms of oral/dental disease such as any carious lesions, active periodontal disease, pulp tissue pathology, occlusal pathology (inclusive of any temporomandibular joint disease), soft and non-dental tissue lesions, and any non-carious hard tissue pathology (inclusive of TW lesions).

Teeth diagnosed as having a *hopeless prognosis* (without any functional/strategic merit) should be considered for extraction. An evaluation of the prognostic outcome of any affected teeth can be based on an assessment of:

- the quantity and quality of the remaining tooth structure
- the periodontal support
- the endodontic status
- the history of the affected tooth.

In relation to worn dentition, traditionally full coverage hard acrylic occlusal splints have been prescribed for cases of generalised TW to ascertain the patient's likely acceptance of the planned occlusal changes (as discussed in Chapter 7). Likewise, removable appliances have been used to provide intra-occlusal clearance (commonly referred to as Dahl appliances, as detailed in Chapters 5 and 11) for cases of localised (anterior) TW. However, given the poor compliance that is often associated with the latter forms of removable appliance together with the continuing evolution of adhesive dental materials technology, the use of adhesive materials may prove to be of great benefit in preventing any further tooth tissue loss, as well as helping to establish the same outcomes as would be expected from the prescription of the aforementioned removable appliances.

Indeed, Briggs et al. have described the use of direct composite resin restorations as an intermediate restorative option amongst patients presenting with TW (*intermediate composite restoration, ICR*).[7] The application of ICR in conjunction with routine preventative measures to manage at-risk sites (to reduce long-term catastrophic damage, particularly where future sporadic bursts of aggressive wear may take place with changes in lifestyle or personal circumstances) is an approach that has been advocated. The role of adhesive materials (as well their limitations for the management of the worn dentition) is discussed at length in Chapter 10.

However, given that the placement of an intermediate composite resin restoration will most likely commit the patient to long-term (and in some cases complex) costly restorative care with associated high maintenance needs,[2] it is pivotal that proper consideration is given to the need to provide *active restorative intervention*, as well as to discuss the means by which this may be most effectively and predictably undertaken.

In general, the decision for implementing active restorative intervention should include a consideration of the following aspects:[5,8]

1) the extent of the TW (grading)
2) the affected surfaces (whether they are involved with providing occlusal contact)
3) the number of teeth affected (localised wear or generalised wear)
4) the rate/progression (speed) of tooth surface loss (taking into consideration the age of the patient)

5) aetiological factors
6) the patient's aesthetic requirements and functional problems.

Restorative intervention is most likely to be prescribed when:

1) there may be significant concerns in relation to the aesthetic zone
2) there is pain and/or discomfort as a result of progressive TW
3) there may be resultant functional impairment
4) consent has been gained following a complete, accurate, balanced, logical, and comprehensive discussion of the risks and benefits of treatment, and the patient has been given the time they need to arrive at a valid decision.

In 2017, as part of the European Consensus Statement on the Management Guidelines for Severe Tooth Wear, Loomans et al.[5] proposed a protocol to aid the process of decision making when planning for care. Accordingly, passive management (inclusive of the prescription of a tailored preventative programme), counselling, and monitoring should be implemented in all cases of pathological TW case regardless of the observed pattern and extent of TW. Amongst cases presenting with no significant concerns (as listed above), no further active intervention may be needed. Patients presenting with insignificant TW for age, which is also likely to be of the quiescent variety, should not be encouraged to subscribe to the need for restorative intervention.

However, where the process of TW is likely to be progressive and the rate of progression present itself as a reason for concern, having established the most probable causative factors and prescribed a preventative programme in accordance under circumstances where the patient may not have complaints, it would be sensible to monitor the success of the preventative regime. If it were ascertained that the rate of TW has reached a quiescent phase, then the options for restorative intervention can be reviewed. Where the choice is taken to defer restorative intervention, vigilant monitoring is advised, with records (for the purposes of monitoring) as discussed above updated every two to three years.

Amongst patients with concerns in relation to aesthetics/function and/or pain, restorative options may be indicated at an earlier point in time. However, they would not normally be advised until stabilisation of the TW pattern had been established.[6]

Where possible, restorative intervention should be:[5]

- deferred for as long as reasonably possible (for the reasons as discussed above)
- undertaken after having attained valid informed consent (ensuring the preparation of suitable clinical records)
- of an additive nature as opposed to subtractive, where the application of restorations that can be provided by minimal intervention that offer the concomitant ability to be readily adjusted, repaired, and removed without sustaining any significant additional tooth tissue loss and/or pulp tissue trauma is granted primary consideration[9–11] (this topic forms the subject of Chapter 9).

Occlusal stabilisation at this stage may also require the provision of some forms of dental prostheses in the event of missing tooth units. The prescription of a suitably designed removable acrylic partial denture may be helpful under such circumstances, as this offers a cost-effective solution that can be readily modified/adjusted if required.

Having stabilised any existing oral disease (by the management of any carious lesions or periodontal pockets, carrying out root canal treatments, prescribing occlusal splints etc.) it is important to evaluate the presence of a successful outcome using established processes. This may include the taking and recording of plaque and bleeding scores, probing depth changes, signs of periapical and pulp tissue resolution, and cessation of the development of carious lesions (often requiring the use of radiographic techniques). This would usually be followed by a reassessment of the original treatment plan and the possible options for managing the worn dentition.

Upon verification of the treatment plan and having ensured the attainment of valid informed consent, the next stage involves the provision of *definitive restorations*. This may include the use of direct and/or indirect materials as well as removable dental prostheses. For further details in relation to the rationale for the selection of a given treatment protocol, the commonly used dental materials, and the techniques employed to permit the technical execution of the clinical stages, see to Chapters 9–13.

Following a period of adaptation and observation, having successfully stabilised the pattern of wear and provided a restored dentition which meets the aesthetic and functional needs of the patient, the need for further *definitive complex restorations* (such as crown, onlay or veneer restoration, especially where the direct approach may have failed to fully meet the functional and aesthetic needs of the patient) may be given due consideration. Treatments at this stage may use techniques that permit the replication of the functional occlusal prescription (as described in Chapter 13) to further improve the likelihood of success with the outcome. With this approach, additive materials can be used to functionally test the patient's adaptation and acceptance of the planned changes prior to the prescription of more complex and costly restorations/restorative materials, which in turn may require some further tooth tissue loss and may be less amenable to repair and/or adjustment in the oral environment.[10]

Careful consideration should be undertaken before the provision of restorations which require the removal of healthy sound tooth tissue, for example full coverage crowns. This can produce further restorative complication and tooth survival issues in the future, and possibly lead to the loss of the tooth when failure of these restorations occurs. Hence the balance between the use of subtractive vs additive techniques requires careful consideration and evaluation.

Edentulous spaces may also be restored using more robust forms of mucosa and tooth-supported removable prostheses, fixed bridgework or dental implants (sometimes in combination). Orthodontic treatment may be required to assist with restorative procedures, such as the uprighting of a tilted tooth, space opening or space closure, or be prescribed to meet the aesthetic needs of the patient, where there may be crowing or spaces present.

Finally, the importance of *monitoring and maintenance* should be emphasised at the outset. In cases where passive management alone has been applied, patients should be regularly reviewed and assessed for disease progression.

Where restorative care may have been provided, restorations (inclusive of their form, aesthetic appearance, and structural and marginal integrity) and the residual dentition (as well as compliance with any prescribed oral appliance(s), such as any post-operative occlusal splints) should be closely observed as failures are likely. Such failures will need to be suitably addressed to maintain the patient's oral health, as well as their functional and aesthetic requirements. The costs associated with any likely longer-term care (as well as any treatment guarantees) should also be clarified at the outset.

8.3   Forming the Aesthetic Prescription for the TW Patient

Where the decision has been taken to undertake restorative rehabilitation, given the complex occlusal, functional, and aesthetic changes that are likely to take place post-restoration it is important to develop an approach that combines predictability in the establishment of the definitive aesthetic prescription with the need to use clinical techniques that permit the opportunity for all concerned parties to reversibly visualise any planned aesthetic changes, gain informed consent, and avoid unrealistic expectations. In practice, this is generally accomplished by the use of one of the following techniques[12]:

- intra-oral mock-up, also referred to as dry-and-try techniques
- digital smile evaluation.

The practical stages associated with the implementation of these techniques are discussed below. Essential background reading in this area is provided in Chapters 3 and 5, where the importance of developing familiarity with the processes involved in the evaluation of the aesthetic zone and the essential concepts in clinical occlusion, respectively, are discussed.

8.3.1   The Intra-oral Mock-Up (Reversible Intra-oral Prototype) Technique

With this method, it is appropriate to start with the selection of a suitable shade of resin composite. The anterior maxillary teeth should ideally be clean and moist with no effort made to prepare the teeth for adhesive bonding. Preferably the mock-up is made on the upper teeth from canine to canine. If necessary, a mock-up can also be made on the anterior teeth.

Where an increase in the length of the central incisor teeth is desired, the width of the tooth should be determined using a dental probe with millimetre markings. Resin composite is then applied to one of the air-dried maxillary central incisor teeth, aiming to achieve a rough length to width ratio of 1.2 : 1. Accordingly, for an average width maxillary central incisor with a width of 8–9 mm, a length of 10–11 mm would be deemed suitable. Where the pre-existing width may present itself as an unsuitable marker, the length of the resting vertical dimension of the patient's face may prove helpful; the length of a central incisor should be approximately one-sixteenth of this dimension. The rest position of the upper lip should also be applied as a useful guide to determining a suitable length.[13] Where a decrease in the length of the selected tooth is desired, a surgical marker pen can be used to mark the desired length to attain the above proportions.

The patient to should then be requested to enunciate the letters 'F' or 'V', with the operator concomitantly observing the relationship between the incisal edge and upper border of the lower lip. Ideally, the incisal edge should be contoured to follow the profile of the upper border of their lower lip, with a constant spatial distance of approximately 3 mm. Having re-established the relationship of the incisal edge to the 'smile arc' during a posed smile, this latter process is repeated at the contra-lateral tooth.

With the aid of a set of wooden spatulas, the relationship between the incisal edges of the maxillary anterior teeth and the inter-pupillary line should be determined. Ideally, parallelism should exist. Where the inter-pupillary line is canted, an alternative reference plane such as the horizon should be utilised.

The profile of the maxillary incisor teeth should next be appraised in a lateral direction. Material should be added or removed to develop a lateral profile that presents itself with two or three planes on the labial (facial) surface and provides an appropriate level lip support.

Attention may now be focussed on contouring the mock-up to crudely reflect the patient's age, sex, personality, and strength index culminating in an ovoid, square, tapering or square-tapering profile. Invariably, the latter will involve the adjustment of the mesial and distal incisal edges. For cases where there may have been considerable loss of incisal edge tissue, thought should be given to the position of the contact area, which should ideally be positioned in the incisal third of the maxillary central incisor tooth, 6 mm coronal to the crestal bone, to develop ultimate papillary infill and the elimination of unwanted black spaces.[14]

For cases where there is a need to alter the width of the maxillary central incisor teeth (such as in the case of diastema closure), resin composite can be added to the inter-proximal surface(s). The width to length ratio may be applied as discussed above. The relationship between the maxillary dental midline and the facial midline should also be appraised; ideally, the discrepancy should be no greater than 2.0 mm.[15]

Often it may be desirable, when the material of choice allows for removal and addition, to omit certain anatomical details such as fissures and surface morphology from the mock-up, as these can easily be incorporated at a later stage. This enables the initial build-up steps to be less complex and time-consuming, with the reduced likelihood of the introduction of occlusal interferences.

Having developed the maxillary central incisor teeth to the desired morphology (or indeed where such teeth may be deemed to be aesthetically acceptable), attention is diverted to the maxillary lateral incisor teeth. Resin may be added in an analogous manner to the above to the incisal edge (assuming an alteration in the length is indicated) such that the incisal edge is placed a couple of millimetres apical to the central incisor, with an overarching aim of developing the profile of the incisal edge in accordance with the patient's smile arc. Thus, in going from the midline, the axial inclination of maxillary anterior teeth should assume a mesial tilt and the mesial contact point should be placed slightly more apical to that formed between the central incisors.

For cases where an alteration in the width of the lateral incisor is desired, the concept of the golden proportion may be applied, as described above. The use of a golden proportion gauge (golden mean gauge) may be helpful with this exercise. The profile of the contra-lateral maxillary lateral incisor should be developed to roughly mimic that of the above. The embrasure space formed between the central and lateral incisors, and indeed that of the canine teeth, should progressively increase in size distally form the midline.

Resin composite may now be added to the maxillary canine teeth, applying the concepts discussed above, with the aim of maintaining symmetry across the midline. The average length of a maxillary canine should be 11–13 mm. In severe TW patients the optimal length sometimes cannot be realised due to compensatory growth of the teeth. An optimal length will then lead to incisors which are clinically too long in relation to the lower lip. Therefore, the intra-oral mock-up will finally determine the length of the teeth.

Attention may now be diverted to the development of the desired gingival aesthetics. Where there is a need to alter this, add resin to simulate the effect of crown lengthening, such that the horizontal levels of the central incisor teeth and canines are in the same plane, with symmetry across the midline and approximately 1 mm apical to that of the lateral incisor.

At this stage, the width of the patient's smile should also be assessed. The presence of black spaces between the cheeks and teeth (negative buccal corridor) may look particularly unaesthetic, thus, if required, resin may be added to the buccal cusp tips of the premolar teeth to assess the effect of reducing this dimension.

Finally, the mandibular teeth should be viewed in relation to the maxillary mock-up. Consideration may be given to adding resin to the mesial surfaces of the lower central incisors, with the aim of attaining a congruent vertical reference with the maxillary centre line, although co-incidence of these planes has been reported to exist amongst 25% of the population only.[16]

Phonetic tests can be of help in determining the height and bucco-palatal width of the anterior teeth. When the patient is asked to enunciate the 'F' sound, typically by counting from 40 to 50, if noisy and imprecise this may be a sign of the need to shorten the length of the maxillary central incisors. In a similar manner, if the palatal surfaces have been over-bulked (which may limit freedom in centric and feel uncomfortable), this will not allow for the effective enunciation of the 'S' sound, which may be elicited by asking the patient to count from 60 to 70.[17]

Having completed the mock-up, it is appropriate to show the proposed changes to the patient using a hand mirror, as well as obtaining high-quality photographs of the mock-up and also considering the taking of a video recording to assess the effects of dynamic aspects such as on their speech. Adjustments can now be readily made as per the patient's desires and further to any dentist–patient discussions by simply adding or removing resin composite.

Once all parties are reasonable satisfied, an over-impression of the mock-up using a suitable form of dental alginate, silicone putty or digital 3D scan should be taken prior to the removal of the mock-up (Figure 8.2).

The above records (including any further information such as occlusal records) should be dispatched to the laboratory with a detailed occlusal prescription, aesthetic prescription, and the photographic records so that an aesthetic and functional diagnostic wax-up may be formed.

8.3.2 Digital Smile Evaluation

With advances in digital photography and information technology software, it has become possible to undertake the process of aesthetic design utilising universally accepted concepts in dental aesthetics, such as those relating to ratios, proportions, tooth position/alignment, shape/form, and colour (Figure 8.3).[17] The process of digital smile evaluation (DSE) requires the taking of an array of full-face photographs using a high-resolution digital camera with a macro lens, followed by the use of a programmed *digital ruler* to carry out assessments of the patient's aesthetic zone.

With the use of this software tool, the clinician is able to display differing tooth proportions (which may be particularly helpful in the case of worn dentition) and thereby:

- simulate the effect of an altered pattern of tooth alignment
- experiment with an array of available differing tooth forms (with the aim of harmonising with the patient's facial features using a library of available differing tooth forms)
- display the effect of changing parameters relating to tooth colour: temperature, brightness, contrast, and saturation.

With these tools, together with input from the patient, the dentist is in a position to design the features of the aesthetic zone.

This information can be used by the dental technician to prepare a diagnostic wax-up, with the added merit of the information being available electronically, as well as the use of CAD technology to fabricate a *virtual wax-up.*

8.4   The Preparation and Evaluation of the Diagnostic Wax-Up

Having determined the choice of restorative material(s), the dental technician will now be in a position to fabricate a diagnostic wax-up to meet the aesthetic and functional demands of the patient. This is usually carried out on a set of accurate casts mounted on a suitable form of dental articulatory. The use of an arcon type of semi-adjustable dental articulator is generally considered acceptable.

From a pragmatic perspective, as discussed in Chapter 6, the concept of a *mutually protected occlusal scheme (MPO)* is frequently used by many practitioners as the occlusal end-point (circumstances permitting) when considering restorative rehabilitation of worn dentition. The presence of a *canine guided/ canine protected occlusion* is also considered to be generally desirable (assuming good health of the canine teeth).[18] This form of occlusal scheme is also relatively easier to accomplish from a technical/clinical perspective when undertaking restorative rehabilitation when compared with the scenario of mandibular guidance provided by a number of posterior teeth on the working side (*group function*).[18]

As part of effective communication, it is imperative that the clinician provides the dental technician with a clear and accurate occlusal prescription, together with any other relevant details as discussed above. The diagnostic wax-up as a standalone is of limited benefit in conveying the proposed aesthetic changes. With the use of a simple technique, the information from the wax-up can be readily transferred into the patient's mouth, allowing them to visualise the proposal intra-orally. This technique is described below.

On receipt of a completed diagnostic wax-up, it should be carefully appraised. If satisfactory, an impression of the wax-up should be taken using a polyvinyl siloxane (PVS) based material or a vacuum-formed polymerizing vinyl chloride (PVC) matrix prepared on a duplicate cast of the wax-up. The patient's teeth should be lightly lubricated using petroleum jelly (concomitantly ensuring that any gross hard tissue undercuts are suitably blocked out) and the chosen shade of provisional crown and bridge resin placed into the impression/matrix, making sure to apply material that crudely conforms to the volume of wax used (avoiding the need to trim away excessive set resin). The impression/matrix is then carefully seated in the mouth; once set, the resin-based material can be carefully trimmed and any refinements required can be made.

Alternatively, the decision can be taken to have a 'clip-on smile' fabricated by the dental laboratory (such as the Snap-on-Smile, by DenMat, USA) or where CAD software has been used, the digital design can be used to mill a model from which a silicone key can be made (DSD Connect, DSD Technology, Romania) and subsequently used to produce an intra-oral mock-up as described above.[17]

The intra-oral mock up derived using the wax-up (sometimes referred to as the 'trial-smile') should be critically appraised, including its aesthetic, occlusal, and phonetic features, as described above. In some cases there may be an indication for the wax-up to be corrected and the process repeated. The use of photographs and/or videos of the mock-up can be beneficial not only to facilitate communication with the laboratory, but to also provide the patient with information that they can take away to make an informed decision about the proposed changes/plan of care, giving them the opportunity and time to discuss matters with their friends/family as well as with the dental operator. The use of videos is also invaluable to establish the dynamic relationships of the lips and perioral tissues to the position of the teeth and visible dento-alveolar profiles.

8.5 Summary and Conclusions

The importance of preparing a logical and appropriate treatment plan to tackle the needs of a patient with TW (which can sometimes be highly complex) cannot be overemphasised. Where possible the use of techniques that permit the patient to provide informed consent should be employed.

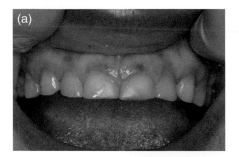
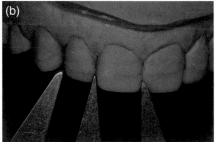
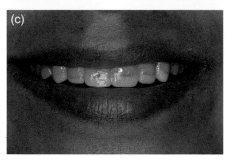

Figure 8.1 Patient with a mock-up done extra-orally in wax and then transferred onto the upper anterior teeth using a putty index and a resin-based temporary crown and bridge material. (a) Pre-operative view of patient's worn upper anterior teeth. (b) Diagnostic wax-up. (c) From an index made from the diagnostic wax-up the prescription is transferred reversibly onto the patient's anterior upper dentition using a temporary crown and bridge material.

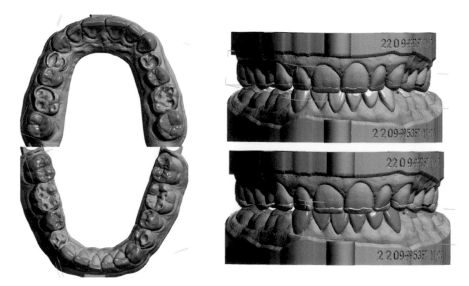

Figure 8.2 Digital mock-up.

Intake   *Preparation*   *Digital wax-up*   *After treatment*

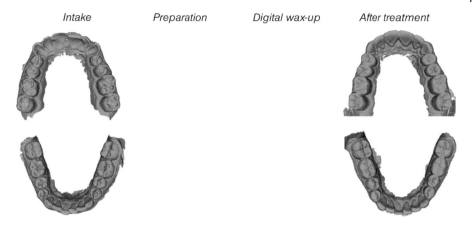

Figure 8.3 Restorations fabricated following digital mock-up using CAD/CAM.

References

1 Newsome, P., Smales, R., and Yip, K. (2010). Oral diagnosis and treatment planning: Part 1. Introduction. *Br. Dent. J.* 213: 15–19.
2 Bartlett, D. (2016). A personal perspective and update on erosive tooth wear – 10 years on: Part 2. Restorative management. *Br. Dent. J.* 221: 167–171.
3 Mehta, S.B., Banerji, S., Millar, B., and Saures-Fieto, J.M. (2012). Current concepts on the management of tooth wear: Part 1. Assessment, treatment planning and strategies for the prevention and passive management of tooth wear. *Br. Dent. J.* 212: 17–27.
4 Watson, M. and Burke, F. (2000). Investigation and treatment of patients with teeth affected by tooth substance loss: a review. *Dent. Update* 27: 175–183.
5 Loomans, B., Opdam, N., Attin, T. et al. (2017). Severe tooth wear: European consensus statement on management guidelines. *J. Adhes. Dent.* 19: 111–119.
6 Johansson, A., Johannson, A., Omar, R., and Carlsson, G. (2008). Rehabilitation of the worn dentition. *J. Oral Rehabil.* 35: 548–566.
7 Briggs, P., Djemal, S., Chana, H., and Kelleher, M. (1998). Young adult patients with established dental erosion – what should be done? *Dent. Update* 25: 166–170.
8 Wetselaar, P. and Lobbezoo, F. (2016). The tooth wear evaluation system: a modular clinical guide for the diagnosis and management planning of worn dentitions. *J. Oral Rehabil.* 43: 69–80.
9 Carvalho, T., Colon, P., Ganss, C. et al. (2015). Consensus report of the European federation of conservative dentistry: erosive tooth wear – diagnosis and management. *Clin. Oral Investig.* 19: 1557–1561.
10 Mehta, S.B., Banerji, S., Millar, B.J., and Saures-Fieto, J.M. (2012). Current concepts in tooth wear management. Part 4. An overview of the restorative techniques and materials commonly applied for the management of tooth wear. *Br. Dent. J.* 212 (4): 169–177.

11 Meyers, I. (2013). Minimum intervention dentistry and the management of tooth wear in general practice. *Aust. Dent. J.* 58: 60–65.

12 Banerji, S., Mehta, S.B., and Ho, C.K. (2017). *Practical Procedures in Aesthetic Dentistry*. Wiley Blackwell.

13 Vig, R. and Brundo, G. (1978). The kinetics of anterior tooth display. *J. Prosthet. Dent.* 39: 502–504.

14 Tarnow, D.P., Magner, A.W., and Fletcher, P. (1992 Dec). The effect of the distance from the contact point to the crest of bone on the presence or absence of the interproximal dental papilla. *J. Periodontol.* 63 (12): 995–996.

15 Johnston, C., Burden, D., and Stevenson, M. (1999). The influence of facial midline discrepancies on dental attractiveness tarings. *Eur. J. Orthod.* 21: 517–522.

16 Miller, E., Bodden, W., and Jamison, H. (1979). A study of the relationship of the dental midline to the facial median line. *J. Prosthet. Dent.* 41: 657–660.

17 Shepperson, A. (2017). Digital smile evaluation. In: *Practical Procedures in Aesthetic Dentistry* (eds. S. Banerji, S.B. Mehta and C.K. Ho), Chapter 2.5, 27–33. Wiley Blackwell.

18 Eliyas, S. and Martin, N. (2013). The management of anterior tooth wear using gold palatal veneers in canine guidance. *Br. Dent. J.* 214: 291–297.

9

Concepts in the Restoration of the Worn Dentition

9.1 Introduction

In general, the placement of restorations for the treatment of tooth wear (TW) may involve the addition of dental materials to the worn surface(s), sometimes only requiring minimal further tooth loss or subtraction (often confined to microscopic changes, utilising the concepts of dental adhesion), or necessitate the use of conventional/traditional placement techniques requiring the need to remove tooth tissue.

The aims of this chapter are to:

- explore the debate between the application of restorations/restorative materials by additive adhesive means versus that of traditional subtractive/conventional means for the management of TW
- provide a brief overview of the essential concepts in dental adhesion
- consider some of the pragmatic aspects involved in helping to promote effective adhesive dentistry.

It is important to note, however, that the application of some forms of adhesively retained restorations will also require some level of planned tooth reduction in order to successfully manage the worn dentition.

9.2 The Additive/Adhesive Approach Versus the Conventional/Subtractive Approach for the Management of Worn Teeth

Conventional restorative techniques (including the prescription of *full and partial coverage crowns*) have been traditionally prescribed for the management of tooth surface loss.[1,2] Such restorations are retained by mechanical features (*retention and resistance form*) that are provided by the processes of undertaking tooth preparation, together with frictional contact formed between the dental cement, the tooth preparation, and restorative material.

However, with progressive developments in adhesive technology, the availability of superior dental materials, improved knowledge and understanding of some of

Practical Procedures in the Management of Tooth Wear, First Edition. Subir Banerji, Shamir Mehta, Niek Opdam and Bas Loomans.
© 2020 John Wiley & Sons Ltd. Published 2020 by John Wiley & Sons Ltd.
Companion website: www.wiley.com/go/banerji/toothwear

the longer-term complications associated with the prescription of convention-ally retained restorations, the general drive towards adopting the approach of restorative treatment by minimal intervention, and further emphasis on the importance of gaining valid informed consent, the use of additive adhesively retained restorations for the management of TW is gaining increasing popularity.[3]

In very simplistic terms, in the case of a worn-down tooth the use of addi-tiveadhesive techniques (involving the chemical bonding of dental material with-out any noteworthy macroscopic tooth reduction) offers the opportunity to *replace/substitute* the lost tooth tissue. However, in the physiological setting (largely as a result of compensatory mechanisms such as dento-alveolar compen-sation),[4] the mere replacement of the lost tissue may lead to unwanted adverse effects by virtue of the restoration now possibly being in *supra-occlusion*.

Whilst in some cases the placement of a restoration in supra-occlusion may be well accepted and serve as a planned course of action (as discussed in Chapters 5 and 11),[5] for patients where the placement of a restoration in supra-occlusion may be feasible the use of adhesive techniques can still be applied to conserva-tively 'bond' certain types of restorations in place. Whilst the latter may necessi-tate some level of tooth preparation, it is likely that the process of adhesively retaining such restorations may alleviate the need for further levels of tooth reduction that may be otherwise needed to retain more extensive restorations (such as full coverage crowns, especially when retained by conventional means).

In the above context, it is relevant to note the views expressed by the European Consensus Statement, Management Guidelines for Severe Tooth Wear,[6] where it is stated:

> When indicated clinically, restorative treatment should wherever possible be 'additive' rather than 'subtractive', as the latter involves the removal of yet more tooth tissue. To protect tooth structure and the pulp, minimum-intervention approaches involving direct, indirect or hybrid techniques should be favoured over approaches comprising very invasive, traditional indirect restorations, which require extensive preparations that sacrifice sound tooth tissue.

This approach was also advocated by the European Federation of Conservative Dentistry for the restorative management of erosive wear.[7]

However, for the treating clinician when planning care for a patient with TW, there are often a plethora of factors to consider when determining the possible treatment options. These factors should be carefully appraised and discussed with the patient and are discussed below.

9.2.1 Tooth Tissue Subtraction

Conventional restorations require the copious removal of sound dental hard tis-sue. It has in fact been estimated that between 62 and 73% of coronal tooth tissue may be lost during the process of preparing a tooth to receive a porcelain fused to metal crown or an all-ceramic crown, whilst the preparation for a tooth to receive an extended veneer may culminate in the loss of 30% of healthy sound tooth tissue.[8]

In contrast, the preparation and placement of *adhesively retained additive restoration* (such as the use of direct resin composite) to replace lost tooth tissue is likely to involve the use of minimal intervention techniques. Indeed, for the successful retention of such restorations (as discussed further below) it will be incumbent for the clinician to preserve as much of the available enamel tissue as possible to help ensure successful adhesion.

In the case of conventional restorations, however, the process of tooth preparation will not only lead to the loss of any residual enamel, but will also reduce the intrinsic strength of the tooth, leading to possible pulpal and/or periodontal complications, as well as potentially compromising the longevity of the restoration and the tooth itself.[9]

The effect of the loss of such levels of tooth tissue when prescribing a conventionally retained restoration in the case of a patient presenting with TW can have deleterious consequences, especially given that the existing dental hard tissues may have already been significantly compromised by the underlying pathology itself.[3]

9.2.2 Risks of Pulp Tissue Trauma

It has been shown that in the process of preparing teeth for ceramic restorations (amongst teeth previously unaffected by dental caries) *irreversible pulp tissue damage* may be sustained. This will most likely be due to the combined effects of the thermal and physical insults sustained during the process of carrying out deep preparations, as well as the effect of bacterial ingress due to possible micro leakage whilst the provisional restoration is in place and/or from the direct toxic effects of the provisional/temporary materials on the pulp tissue.[9,10] Such an effect on the pulp tissues may not only lead to the development of acute pulpitis, but also result in tooth discoloration, chronic sensitivity, and/or the subsequent need for either endodontic treatment and/or an extraction as a result of irreversible pulp necrosis.[9]

The risks of full coverage restorations on pulp tissue health have been well documented. Saunders and Saunders in 1998 reported 19% of crowned teeth amongst a Scottish subpopulation to show radiographic signs of peri-radicular disease,[11] whilst in 1984 Bergenhotlz and Nyman determined a 9% risk of developing endodontic complications following periodontal and prosthetic treatment of patients with advanced periodontal disease.[12]

Although it has since been suggested that a more realistic estimation of the loss of vitality following the preparation and provision of a crown restoration is in the order of 4–8% in the 10 years following active treatment,[13] in the case of a tooth affected by the aetiological factors that lead to pathological wear, the risks of endodontic complications may indeed be heightened as the pulp tissues may have already been stressed by the cumulative insults sustained from the effects of the aetiological factors that cause TW. Furthermore, iatrogenic pulp exposure is perhaps more likely to be encountered amongst teeth which have been severely affected by the process of wear during the process of carrying out tooth preparation involving the occlusal surface of the affected tooth, by virtue of the pulp chamber being closer to the occlusal surface of the affected tooth.

The risks of pulp tissue complications are likely to be minimal for restorations that do not require any noteworthy macroscopic tooth tissue loss, as discussed further in Chapter 10.

9.2.3 Need for Appropriate Operator Skill and the Availability of the Desired Quantity and Quality of Residual Tooth Tissue(s)

The process of providing a conventionally retained restoration requires the treating clinical to execute precise tooth preparation to deliver the necessary retention and resistance forms, as well as to ensure the required level of intra-occlusal clearance to effectively accommodate the desired amount of restorative material. Failure to do this may have a marked impact on the longevity, durability, aesthetic, and functional outcomes of the definitive restoration.

However, in the case of a worn dentition, the absence of a desirable quantity of dental hard tissue may render the attainment of the desired tooth preparation form highly challenging. In some cases, this may necessitate an alternative treatment approach (sometimes requiring a compromise to be made, for instance the use of an alternative material), whilst in other cases there may be the need for (sometimes complex) *pre-restorative treatment*. This may include periodontal surgery, orthodontic treatment, elective endodontics (that may also involve the placement of a post-retained core),[3] or compromises to be reached in relation to matters such as the dental aesthetics. These aspects are discussed in further detail in Chapters 11–14. In general, however, it has been suggested that where there may be less than 5 mm of coronal height, consideration should be given to the need for surgical crown lengthening to apically reposition the gingival margin.[14]

In the case of adhesively retained restorations, there is also a need for good operator skill/knowledge and experience. However, of paramount importance to success are the presence of a copious quantity of high-quality tooth enamel and the need to provide good moisture control during the stage of carrying out adhesive bonding. These matters are discussed further below. Nonetheless, in the presence of unfavourable circumstances, may deter the recommendation for an adhesively retained restoration. This aspect is discussed further with reference to case examples in Chapter 13.

9.2.4 Need for Provisional Restorations

The prescription of traditional (non-chairside, laboratory fabricated) conventionally retained restorations will incur the need for *provisional indirect restoration(s)*. The latter will serve to maintain functional and aesthetic form whilst the definitive restoration(s) are being fabricated, as well as to secure and maintain oral health. Provisional restorations will not, however, be required when placing direct resin composite additions. The need for such provisional restorations will undoubtedly add to the overall treatment cost, complexity of care, the risk of developing further unwanted effects such as the development of pulp tissue and periodontal pathology, as well as to the overall treatment time.

The prescription of appropriate provisional restorations can, however, offer the merit of allowing the clinician to trial planned functional, occlusal and aesthetic changes;[14] the established features may then be 'copied' into the definitive restorations (as discussed further in Chapters 5 and 13). This can help to enhance the overall predictability of the outcome.[3]

However, in the event of a minimally invasive protocol being adopted, such as with the addition of resin composite, given that restorations may be readily adjusted (by addition or subtraction) or indeed removed without any significant harm being sustained, this will allow the operator the opportunity to test drive planned changes with far reduced risk.[3] In contrast, the loss of tooth tissue that will take place as a consequence of providing a conventionally retained restoration will be of the irreversible variety. The latter may pose a significant clinical dilemma (as well as potential medico-legal complications) in the event of the patient being unable to accept/tolerate the aesthetic and/or functional outcome.

9.2.5 Treatment Cost/Time Costs

The associated (and often high) treatment fees for the rehabilitation of a patient with TW can sometimes serve as a barrier to the provision of care.

There is often some debate about the cost of the application of adhesively retained restorations versus that of conventional restorations. This is further compounded by differences in the due reimbursement systems between various countries around the world. As discussed in Chapter 11, the direct application of resin composite is often used to treat TW (especially involving the anterior teeth). Whilst good short- to medium-term survival rates are found with the use of such restorations,[15] longer-term success may be hampered by the need for copious maintenance and remedial therapy.[14] The latter may have financial implications for the patient.

Although the prescription of resin composite has been estimated to be approximately three times less than that for indirectly fabricated restorations in the initial setting,[3] given perhaps the (general) lower short- to medium-term maintenance needs for more robust/durable dental materials (such as full coverage crowns), the latter may ultimately culminate in being of relatively less of a financial burden as well as being more time-effective (with the reduced need for what sometimes may prove to be lengthy and undesirable unplanned visits to ensure ongoing function).

Indeed, it has been suggested by Bartlett[14] that the use of crowns may be considered a reasonable option where erosion is significantly involved with the aetiology of TW. However, where severe bruxism may be a major causative factor for the observed pathology, there is no guarantee that any restoration will be successful. Accordingly, crowns may not serve as an appropriate form of intervention. Where a crown restoration is to be prescribed, it is the view of the authors that for patients with a primarily erosive cause it is possible to consider all ceramic crowns, but for patients with an underlying aetiology of bruxism, metal ceramic crowns and, when possible, full metal (gold) crowns may serve as a better treatment option.[14]

9.2.6 Contingency Planning

Whilst there is likely to be ongoing maintenance needs with the prescription of direct resin composite restorations to treat TW[14] (where higher levels of minor failure can be expected with such restorations), the failures encountered are often amenable to repair, or at least likely to enable the prescription of an indirect (and sometimes conventionally retained) restoration.[16] Indeed, for some patients adhesive restorations may initially be prescribed as medium-term/interim restorations,[3] where eventually, having established acceptance of the planned aesthetic and functional changes, thought may be given to the substitution of the interim restorations with more robust restorative materials (sometimes involving the use of conventional techniques). This may also have the benefit of spreading the financial cost of rehabilitation of the worn dentition with the added benefit of being able to provide indirect restorations in a more predictable and manageable sequence. However, recent research reports confirmed the reliability of direct composites for treatment of TW, whilst indirect composites, although more wear resistant, seem to result in more bulk fractures.

Whilst there is some limited evidence to support the role of conventional restorations reliant on preparation resistance and retention form as offering superior levels of longevity when compared to minimally invasive adhesive restorations in the medium to longer term,[16] the same evidence also highlights the likely longer-term failures associated with conventionally retained longer term to be of the catastrophic variety, where endodontic treatment or a dental extraction may prove to be the next step in the restorative cycle. Consequently, contingency planning with conventional restorations may prove to be far more challenging (if indeed at all possible).[16]

9.2.7 The Aesthetic Outcome

The placement of full coverage restorations has the merit of offering the operator further control of the aesthetic outcome. In contrast, when simply bonding material to the tooth surface(s) without undertaking any macroscopic tooth reduction, there is the heightened risk of an aesthetic disparity arising between the tooth and the restorative material. In some cases, this effect can be masked by extending the restorative material across the whole facial surface, but this can lead to an undesirable tooth form/emergence profile, which may impact on the aesthetic outcome as well as hamper good oral health (e.g. where a restoration may result in an alteration of the emergence profile of a tooth, resulting in further plaque entrapment, gingivitis, gingival recession or periodontitis).[8]

It is therefore important to have a clear discussion with the patient during the stages of planning care. There is some evidence to suggest that when patients are adequately informed (in relation to the treatment being prescribed in the aesthetic zone), they may opt for the more conservative option using aesthetic tooth-coloured alternatives as opposed to more destructive techniques required to accommodate ceramic restorations, where survival of the tooth may be appreciated to be of greater benefit than the survival or indeed aesthetic outcome of the restoration.[17] The latter study also showed that patients do not perceive porcelain restorations to necessarily be more aesthetic than resin composite restorations.[17]

The concept of *pragmatic aesthetics* is often applied under such circumstances, where for many patients minor aesthetic compromise may be acceptable in exchange for tooth conservation or the need for invasive periodontal surgery.[18]

9.3 Concepts in Dental Adhesion

There are a large number of adhesive bonding systems in the marketplace. In general, an adhesive system will comprise:

- an etching agent
- a primer
- bonding agent

Each of the above will have a role of bonding to enamel and dentine. However, for descriptive purposes, the topics of *enamel bonding* and *dentine bonding* will be considered separately.

9.3.1 Enamel Bonding

The process of etching enamel is usually performed using 37% orthophosphoric acid, with a typical pH value of 0.5. The latter agent not only demineralizes the hydroxyapatite structure in enamel, but also acts on the dentine tissues, although with lesser uniformity. The effect of the etchant on the dental hard tissues is to create pores in the micro-structure, allowing the subsequent permeation of resin of flowable consistency through these pores, forming a micro-mechanical lock, commonly referred to as *resin tags*.

An alternative way to produce this etching pattern is to apply acid monomers, as in self-etching and universal bonding systems. Adhesion using the etch-and-rinse technique with phosphoric acid is generally the most reliable for enamel and is therefore recommended for most TW cases.

Use of the acid etchant leads to dissolving (etch-and-rinse) or modification (self-etch) of the *smear layer*, which is a thin layer composed of debris formed by the process of cavity preparation. With etch-and-rinse systems this smear layer is removed (rinsed away) whilst in self-etching systems acid monomers etch the smear layer and the surface, resulting in monomer salts being part of the adhesive layer. The means by which this layer is managed during the adhesive protocol can influence the bond strength attained, as discussed below.

Typical shear bond strengths of resin composite to phosphoric acid etched enamel appear to be in the range of 20 MPa, which is considered to be sufficient to resist the stresses produced by polymerisation shrinkage of resin composites,[19] and supersedes the bond strengths that can be attained by contemporary systems with dentine. In some cases of TW severe loss of enamel tissue can be seen. However, the presence of a peripheral rim of enamel often termed the 'enamel ring of confidence' can provide the clinician with the security of knowing the likelihood of attaining an appropriate circumferential margin seal. Such areas can often be seen amongst patients presenting with severe maxillary anterior palatal surface wear, where the existence of enamel patency at the gingival margin is thought to be accounted for by the protective influence offered by the surrounding gingival cervicular fluid.

Microscopically, the effect of etching enamel with phosphoric acid will lead to the formation of various *etching patterns*, which are commonly described as being Type I, II or III. A *Type I* pattern results from the loss of inter-prismatic enamel, whilst as part of the *Type II* pattern, intra-prismatic enamel is observed to be removed instead. The *Type III* pattern displays a combination of the patterns seen with Types I and II. It has been suggested that the Type II pattern is ideal for the process of resin bonding.[20]

The *orientation of the enamel prisms* has also been shown to have a marked effect on the enamel bond tensile strength, whereby composite resin when bonded parallel to the enamel prism results in the development of higher micro-tensile bond strengths as opposed to the process of bonding perpendicular to enamel prisms.[21]

The process of *selective enamel etching* is also sometimes described in the literature.[22] As part of this protocol, the enamel margins are etched with phosphoric acid, with the dentine tissues being spared from the etchant. This method has been suggested when using self-etching or universal adhesives to result in enamel margins that are less vulnerable to staining, as well as offering the potential to protecting the dentine bond by the formation of an enamel–composite interface.[23]

9.3.2 Dentine Bonding

It is generally accepted that dentine bonding is less predictable than enamel bonding. However, as many patients with severe TW may display copious levels of dentine exposure, the importance of attaining an effective bond with this tissue is of key importance to adhesive restorative success.

The relative difficulty with bonding to dentine is primarily accounted for by:[24]

- higher water content (approximately 10%)
- the structural heterogeneity of this tissue (with the presence of a tubular arrangement)
- higher organic content (collagen fibres by approximately 40%), as opposed to the heavily mineralised, prismatic, hydrophobic nature of enamel
- the long-term stability of the bond developed between dentine tissue and the adhesive luting agents
- the intra-pulpal fluid pressure generated via the vital pulp, resulting in continuous risk of moist surfaces that may jeopardise adequate bonding.

Bonding to dentine usually involves three stages: conditioning (provided by the effect of the application of the acid etchant), priming, and bonding. The process of *conditioning* either removes or modifies the smear layer and is discussed further below.

There is a plethora of differing dentine bonding systems available in the marketplace, but in general the current bonding agents may be classed as being:

- *etch-and-rinse* (also termed *etch and bond* or *total etch*): these involve the simultaneous etching of enamel and dentine, followed by a post-conditioning rinse to remove the smear layer)

- *self-etch*: these incorporate both a primer and an acid and may be classified further into (i) those with strong etching potential and (ii) those with mild etching potential
- *universal systems*: these incorporate both a primer and an acid and offer the opportunity to use the system in self-etch mode as well as etch and rinse mode.

Self-etching systems may seem appealing to many clinicians, as their use offers pragmatic (time- and effort-saving) benefits. However, there is evidence from a systematic review to suggest that the efficacy offered by some types of these systems, especially strong etching adhesives (as measured by their function to retain restorations amongst non-retentive cavities, such as Class V lesions), may be less than optimal.[25] This may be because polymer salts resulting from strong self-etching systems are more soluble, leading to deterioration of the adhesive layer in the long term. Whilst this level of pH in mild self-etching systems may be sufficiently low to etch the dentine surface and permit bonding, the pH of these products is weaker than the pH of commonly used preparations of phosphoric acid. Consequently, the bond strength with the enamel tissues using self-etch systems is usually weaker, and is the reason for many believing that the process of using separate etch followed by prime and bonding or total etch is the gold standard when etching enamel.[26] However, mild self-etch systems, especially two-step systems, show comparable results in clinical Class V cases, and these adhesives also belong to the contemporary gold standard.[27]

It has been suggested by Burke[28] that amongst cases of TW with copious dentine exposure, with little remaining enamel, and cases where the cavity preparation will not offer adequate mechanical retention and resistance form (thus, where the role of dentine bonding may be critical to the survival of the restoration), the use of etch and rinse systems should be preferred, at least until further substantial evidence emerges to support the use of self-etching systems under such circumstances.

9.3.2.1 Primers

Non-etching primers are used in adhesive systems that employ phosphoric acid for the necessary conditioning of the enamel. They are adhesion-promoting agents with a bifunctional molecular structure comprising a monomer component with hydrophobic properties that has an affinity towards any exposed collagen present in the dentinal tubules and a hydrophobic monomer that can form a chemical link with the resin present in the bond. This results in the formation of a *hybrid layer* between the tooth surface, primer and resin-bonding agent. All of these dentin primers also contain a solvent, either ethanol or acetone, enabling the primer to enter the demineralised structure resulting from etching with phosphoric acid. A disadvantage of etch-and-rinse systems is that etching combined with (over)drying may result in a collagen collapse, preventing impregnation of the primer and subsequent bonding in the demineralised zone. An ethanol-based primer, often also containing water, may compensate for this effect as it acts as a rewetting agent. Primers with acetone as solvent are especially sensitive for collagen collapse and for those systems a wet bonding technique is mandatory. However, such a technique may be very difficult to standardise and therefore it is a likely explanation for the postoperative sensitivity that especially these generations of adhesives based on acetone have been notorious for.

The agent hydroxyethyl methacrylate (HEMA) is generally present in most primers, as well as solvents such as ethanol or acetone to help displace water from the dentine surface. On solvent evaporation, porosities are left in the dentine substrate, which will enhance the adhesive bond.

Other bifunctional monomers used in commercially available bonding systems include 4-methacryloxydecyl trimelliate (4-META) and 2-methacryloxyethyl phenyl hydrogen phosphate (phenyl-P). The best functioning functional monomer seems to be 10-methacrlyoxydecyl dihydrogen phosphate (10-MDP), which offers a chemical bond to calcium in dentin, including nanolayering, which enhances the quality of dentine bonding in the long term. The 10-MDP monomer was patented by Kuraray for many years but recently other brands have been introduced, although there are significant differences in the quality of the monomers between the various brands.[29]

Self-etching primers contain the above-mentioned monomers but also include acidic monomers for dissolving hydroxyapatite. The solvent is always water, which is more difficult to remove compared to ethanol and acetone, and requires a more accurate drying process from the clinician.

The advantage of self-etching for dentin bonding is that the demineralised zone always contains monomers. Problems such as collagen collapse do not exist and self-etching systems are well known for their low incidence of post-operative sensitivity.

9.3.2.2 Bonding Resins

The *bonding resins* most commonly used are based on bisphenol A-glycidyl methacrylate (Bis-GMA) or urethane dimethacrylate (UDMA). As these monomers are inherently viscous as well as being hydrophobic, they are usually diluted in hydrophilic monomers of lower viscosity to improve their wettability. The *diluents* most commonly used include HEMA and triethylene-glycol dimethacylate (TEG-DMA). Functional monomers such as 10-MDP are also often incorporated in bonding agents.

Those bonding systems that do not use a separate primer require a solvent such as water, acetone or ethanol to be included. As these solvents need to be evaporated, leaving behind porosities in the bonding layer, these systems have been shown to be clinically inferior compared to those systems that apply primers and bonding in sequential steps.[28]

In a well-functioning bonding system, bonding resins will enter the porosities created by the removal of the smear layer and the demineralisation of the surface layer of the hydroxyapatite crystal by the process of acid etching and therefore create resin tags, which provide micro-mechanical retention, as well as by penetration of the dentinal tubules and the formation of a chemical bond with the primer, resulting in the development of the hybrid layer.

Histological variations in dentine such as those that occur with the process of ageing (culminating in a hyper-mineralised substrate by the processes of the sclerosis of dentine as well as the formation of reparative and reactionary dentine) or those that occur as dentine approaches the pulp (resulting in a 'wetter' bonding surface with a concomitant increase in the number of tubules) also compound the predictability of adhesion of resin composite to dentine. Indeed, significantly weaker bond strengths have been described that occur between hyper-mineralised dentine when compared to normal dentine with the formation of thin resin tags and the absence of a hybrid layer.[26]

9.3.3 The Classification of the Available Bonding Agents

It is common to refer to bonding agents by their *generation of introduction*. The first three generations are perhaps best considered as being obsolete. The *fourth-generation* (also termed Type 1) self-etching adhesives are based on a three-step total etch technique and are regarded as the gold standard in contemporary dental practice, together with the sixth generation.[27] A fourth-generation adhesive includes the stage of applying a separate etchant (37% orthophosphoric acid) to sound enamel for 20 seconds and dentine for 10–15 seconds (total etch technique), followed by complete rinsing away with water. This process removes the smear layer. This is followed by the placement of a bespoke primer, preferably with ethanol, to avoid collagen collapse. Gentle drying of the primer is often advocated to permit solvent evaporation, followed by placement of the bonding resin.

Examples of a commercially available Type 1 fourth-generation bonding system include Optibond FL (Kerr), All-Bond 2 (Bisco), and Adper Scotchbond MP (3 M ESPE). Bonds obtained with fourth-generation systems are longer lasting than successor products.

Fifth-generation (Type 2) systems are characterised by a two-bottle process comprising a separate etchant that helps to remove the smear layer and a combined prime and bond. Commonly used examples include OptiBond Solo PLus (Kerr), Prime and Bond NT (Denstply-Detrey), and Excite (Ivoclar, Vivadent). The use of these agents carries the risk of desiccating the collagen layer after the process of rising and drying the etchant. There is a need to avoid the collapse of the collagen scaffold (by excessive drying) in order to produce adequate bond strength. There is therefore the need to wet or moisten dentine, which is typically achieved by the blotting of dentine with a moistened cotton wool pledget. Variations in the latter by different clinicians may affect the efficacy of the bond strength developed. The use of these systems, especially those that are acetone-based, may result in post-operative sensitivity when wet bonding is not applied properly.

The *sixth and seventh generations* (Types 3 and 4, respectively) differ in the way in which the smear layer is modified. Whilst they aim to attain a similar type of bond to enamel, they do not remove the smear layer in the same manner as their predecessors do, but rather penetrate the smear layer, dissolve it, and incorporate it into the final adhesive interface.[25] The two generations differ in that the seventh generation of bonding agents has a single-bottle system, with combined etchant, primer and bond, whist the sixth generation has a two-bottle arrangement with a combined etch and primer and a separate bonding resin. Sixth-generation (together with fourth-generation) adhesives are considered to be gold standard adhesives.

Commercial examples of sixth-generation agents include Clearfil SEBond (Kuraray) and One Coat SE Bond (Coltene, Whaledent), whilst popular seventh-generation agents include Adper L-Pop Prompt (3M ESPE), G Bond (GC), and iBond (Heraeus Kultzer). It has been shown that the bond strengths developed with seventh-generation agents are weaker than those of fourth- and sixth-generation agents, thereby increasing the risk of restorative failure by the process of breakdown of the adhesive interface.

Eighth-generation or *universal adhesives* can be delivered as separate primer and bonding or combined primer and bonding. The clinician has the choice of applying phosphoric acid etching as either selective or total etching. Universal adhesives also contain silane coupling agents for bonding to restorative materials. These adhesives claim to simplify bonding procedures but long-term clinical results are not available yet. Commercial examples of eighth-generation adhesives include Clearfil Universal Bond and Scotchbond universal.

In view of the increasing generations of adhesives it is perhaps better to classify these in terms of one-, two- or three-step adhesive protocols.

9.4 Some Pragmatic Considerations when Attempting to Apply Adhesive Techniques to the Management of TW

From a clinical perspective, to attain a desirable bond between the adhesive dental material, the bonding agent, and the worn tooth, it may be appropriate consider some of the following aspects:

- *Appropriate isolation techniques* should be used to provide a moisture and saliva contaminant-free environment that is conducive to optimal resin bonding. Ideally a dental dam is applied, however, especially when the TW extends towards the gingival margins on lingual and buccal surfaces, certain techniques (like the direct shaping by occlusion (DSO) technique, see Chapter 14) preclude the use of rubberdam. In these cases, meticulous placement of wedges and matrices combined with devices like Optragate (Ivoclar Vivadent) (Figure 9.1), cotton wool rolls, suction, and the assistance of a chairside nurse enable moisture control.
- *Preparation of the enamel margin*: Whilst some operators elect to remove any unsupported enamel tissue (using Brown silicone rubber points, discs or ultrasonic instrumentation), for a worn tooth in particular it is imperative to preserve as much enamel at the cavity margins as possible, where any macroscopic preparation, including bevel placement, may take place at the expense of compromising the likely marginal seal.

  For anterior teeth, *bevelling* of the facial/ buccal enamel margins (by 0.5–1.0 mm) has been advocated by some clinicians (where a suitable amount and quality of residual enamel may be present, especially of the *aprismatic variety*) as it exposes enamel rods transversely, thereby presenting a greater surface area for etching and bonding. It is also thought to provide a more effective etching pattern.

There does, however, appear to be a variation in opinion as to the size and form of the bevel, with some operators advocating the use of a two-part bevel, with an initial smaller bevel (perhaps less than 1.0 mm) at 45° followed by a wider diffused scalloped bevel that is less steep but slightly longer in width to further enhance the transition between the resin composite material and the tooth.

Bevelling is perhaps best achieved using a flame-shaped finishing bur or a fine diamond bur. In general, the use of diamond burs will have the effect of 'grinding' the enamel, resulting in a thicker smear layer. In contrast, tungsten carbide flutes will provide the effect of 'cutting' the surface, culminating in a cleaner, less smeared surface for etching.

On the *palatal/lingual surfaces*, as aesthetics is less critical, the use of a longer bevel has little merit. A butt-joint margin is generally also preferable at these locations on account of the variation in the enamel prism arrangement seen. In the opinion of the authors and in their clinical practice bevelling of the enamel is seldom carried out.

- The use of air abrasion of the enamel following cavity preparation and prior to etching is beneficial and helps to remove any peripheral staining and assist with the provision of micromechanical retention.
- It is good practice to ensure the complete removal of etchant agent as well as any dissolved calcium phosphate precipitates in order to produce a clean etched field, concomitantly making sure that the air and water syringes used are free from contaminants (especially compressor oil). It is useful to hold the high-volume aspirator tip next to the tooth after the etch rinse and drying process has taken place. This ensures that the surfaces remain dry prior to the application of the next step.
- Optical magnification can be used to make sure that agents are applied uniformly across the entire adhesive interface. It is also important to avoid the excessive pooling of bonding agents.
- It is imperative to pay close attention to the timing and mode of application of the various agents used as part of the adhesive protocol.
- Light curing units should also be carefully monitored as they may display a progressive decline in function over time and will need regular testing. When using light curing it is good practice to bring the light-curing tip close to the surface and then, whilst holding it rigidly, commence the activation process. This will help ensure that the materials receive the full-recommended polymerisation process.

9.5 Summary and Conclusions

In summary, it is imperative to ensure that all treatment options are appropriately presented and discussed, and as part of doing so longer-term care needs should also be appraised. However, where possible a minimally invasive protocol should be applied for the management of a worn dentition. Appropriate records should be maintained of all discussions. It is also necessary for the contemporary dental practitioner to have a sound working knowledge of the concepts in dental adhesion and the materials used to ensure an optimal outcome.

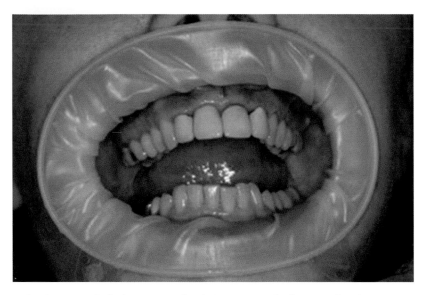

Figure 9.1 Patient with the lips retracted with Optragate to facilitate tooth isolation.

References

1 Malkoc, M., Sevimay, M., and Yaprak, E. (2009). The use of zirconium and feldspathic porcelain in the management of the severely worn dentition: a case report. *Eur. J. Dent.* 3: 75–80.
2 Nam, J. and Tokutomi, H. (2015). Using zirconia-based prosthesis in complete-mouth reconstruction treatment for worn dentition with altered vertical dimension of occlusion. *Prosthet. Dent.* 113: 81–85.
3 Mehta, S.B., Banerji, S., Millar, B., and Saures-Fieto, J.M. (2012). Current concepts on the management of tooth wear: Part 3: Active restorative care 2: The management of generalised tooth wear. *Br. Dent. J.* 212 (3): 121–127.
4 Berry, D. and Poole, D. (1976). Attrition: possible mechanisms of compensation. *J. Oral Rehabil.* 30: 201–206.
5 Poyser, N., Porter, R., Briggs, P. et al. (2005). The Dahl concept: past, present and future. *Br. Dent. J.* 198: 669–676.
6 Loomans, B., Opdam, N., Attin, T. et al. (2017). Severe tooth wear: European consensus statement on management guidelines. *J. Adhes. Dent.* 19: 111–119.
7 Carvalho, T., Colon, P., Ganss, C. et al. (2015). Consensus report of the European federation of conservative dentistry: erosive tooth wear – diagnosis and management. *Clin. Oral Investig.* 19: 1557–1561.
8 Edelhoff, D. and Sorensen, J. (2002). Tooth structure removal associated with various preparation designs for anterior teeth. *J. Prosthet. Dent.* 87 (5): 503–509.
9 Alani, A., Kelleher, M., Hemmings, K. et al. (2015). Balancing the risks and benefits associated with cosmetic dentistry – a joint statement by UK specialist dental societies. *Br. Dent. J.* 218: 543–547.

10 Fleisch, L., Cleaton-Jones, P., Forbes, M. et al. (1984). Pulpal response to a bisacrylplastic (Protemp) temporary crown and bridge material. *J. Oral Pathol.* 13: 622–631.

11 Saunders, W. and Saunders, E. (1998). Prevalence of periradicular periodontitis associated with crowned teeth in the adult Scottish subpopulation. *Br. Dent. J.* 185: 137–140.

12 Bergenholtz, G. and Nyman, S. (1984). Endodontic complications following periodontal and prosthetic treatment of patients with advanced periodontal disease. *J. Periodontal* 55: 63–68.

13 Whitworth, J., Walls, G., and Wassell, R. (2002). Crowns and extra-coronal restorations; endodontic complications: the pulp, the root-treated tooth and the crown. *Br. Dent. J.* 192: 315–327.

14 Bartlett, D. (2016). A personal perspective and update on erosive tooth wear – 10 years on: Part 2: Restorative management. *Br. Dent. J.* 221: 167–171.

15 Loomans Kreulen, C.M., Huijs-Visser, H.E.C.E., Sterenborg, B.A.M.M. et al. (2018). Clinical performance of full rehabilitations with direct composite in severe tooth wear patients: 3 5 years results. *J. Dent.* 70: 97–103. https://doi.org/10.1016/j.jdent.2018.01.001.

16 Smales, R. and Berekally, T. (2007). Long-term survival of direct and indirect restorations placed for the treatment of advanced tooth wear. *Eur. J. Prosthodont. Restor. Dent.* 15 (1): 2–6.

17 Nalbandian, S. and Millar, B.J. (2009). The effect of veneers on cosmetic improvement. *Br. Dent. J.* 207: E3.

18 Burke, F.J.T., Kelleher, M., Wilson, N., and Bishop, K. (2011). Introducing the concept of pragmatic esthetics with special reference to the treatment of tooth wear. *J. Esthet. Restor. Dent.* 23 (5): 277–293.

19 Gilpatrick, R., Ross, J., and Simonsen, R. (1991). Resin-to-enamel bond strengths with various etching times. *Quintessence Int.* 22: 47–49.

20 Van Noort, R. (2008). *Introduction to dental materials*, 3e. Mosby Elsevier.

21 Carvalho, R.M., Santiago, S.L., Fernandes, C.A.O. et al. (2000). Effects of prism orientation on tensile strength of enamel. *J. Adhes. Dent.* 2: 251–257.

22 Peumans, M., de Munck, J., van Landuyt, K. et al. (2010). Eight-year clinical evaluation of a 2-step self-etch adhesive with and without selective enamel etching. *Dent. Mater.* 26: 1176–1184.

23 Burke, F.J.T. (2012). Selective enamel etching. Don't throw away your phosphoric acid, yet! *Dent. Update* 39: 380.

24 Green, D. and Banerjee, A. (2011). Contemporary adhesive bonding: bridging the gap between research and clinical practice. *Dent. Update* 38: 439–450.

25 Pneumans, M., Kanumilli, P., de MUnck, J. et al. (2005). Clinical effectiveness of contemporary dental adhesives: a systematic review of clinical trials. *Dent. Mater.* 21: 864–881.

26 Burke, F.J.T., Lawson, A., Green, D.J.B., and Mackenzie, L. (2017). What's new in dentine bonding?: universal adhesives. *Dent. Update* 44: 328–340.

27 Peumans, M., De Munck, J., Mine, A., and Van Meerbeek, B. (2014 Oct). Clinical effectiveness of contemporary adhesives for the restoration of non-carious cervical lesions. A systematic review. *Dent. Mater.* 30 (10): 1089–1103.

28 Burke, F.J.T. (2014). Information for patients undergoing treatment for tooth wear with resin composite restorations placed at an increased occlusal vertical dimension. *Dent. Update* 41: 28–38.

29 Yoshihara, K., Nagaoka, N., Okihara, T. et al. (2015 Dec). Functional monomer impurity affects adhesive performance. *Dent. Mater.* 31 (12): 1493–1501.

Further Reading

Donaldson, L.F. (2006). Understanding pulpitis. *J. Physiol.* 573 (Pt 1): 2–3. https://doi.org/10.1113/jphysiol.2006.110049PMCID: PMC1779693.

Fradeani, M., Barducci, G., and Bacherini, L. (2016). Esthetic regabilitation of a worn dentition with a minimally invasive prosthetic procedure (MIPP). *Int. J. Esthet. Dent.* 11 (1): 16–34.

Opdam, N., Skupien, J.A., Kreulen, C.M. et al. (2016). Case report: a predictable technique to establish occlusal contact in extensive direct composite resin restorations: the DSO-technique. *Oper. Dent.* 41 (S7): S96–S108.

10

Dental Materials: An Overview of Material Selection for the Management of Tooth Wear

10.1   Introduction

There is a plethora of dental materials that can be used to restore the worn denti-tion.[1] Whilst it is beyond the scope of this text to consider the chemical composi-tion and physical properties of each of these materials in depth, it is vital that the clinician is familiar with the role of the differing materials that may be used to restore the worn dentition. The latter is further supported by the absence of any decisive evidence to substantially favour the use of one material over another[2] or a specific technique of material application (direct or indirect),[2] where some may prove to be more suitable for the management of certain patterns and/or causes of tooth wear (TW), for instance, where the patient may display a tendency towards bruxism or parafunctional activity.[3]

According to Poyser et al.[4] the position within the dental arch of each worn tooth, and the quantity of remaining tooth tissue, will also help determine the most appropriate form of restoration. Whilst conventional restorations have been used historically (such as conventional cast gold onlays, partial and full veneer crowns, or metallo-ceramic crowns), with advances in adhesive dentistry and material properties several other options have also become available. These include the use of:

- direct composite resin restorations
- indirect composite resin restorations
- cast adhesive alloys (metal palatal veneers and metal adhesive onlays)
- adhesive ceramic restorations
- adhesive polymer ceramics.

This chapter provides an overview of the dental materials listed above together with the restorations that are most frequently recommended for the treatment of the worn dentition (including conventionally retained restorations, as eluded to in Chapter 9). It will also include an appraisal of the available contemporary data in relation to the clinical performance of dental restorations fabricated from these materials, especially given that the active management of TW will unfortunately commit the patient to lifelong maintenance. It is imperative that this is effectively communicated and understood from the outset as part of

Practical Procedures in the Management of Tooth Wear, First Edition. Subir Banerji, Shamir Mehta, Niek Opdam and Bas Loomans.
© 2020 John Wiley & Sons Ltd. Published 2020 by John Wiley & Sons Ltd.
Companion website: www.wiley.com/go/banerji/toothwear

gaining informed consent. Clear, complete, and contemporaneous dental records should be kept accordingly.

It is perhaps also relevant to note that there is very limited scientific data concerning the success/survival of conventionally retained fixed indirect prosthodontic restorations to treat TW.

10.2   The Use of Resin Composite to Treat TW

Resin composite restorations may be fabricated directly (chair side) or indirectly (laboratory fabricated).

10.2.1   Direct Composite Resin Restorations

Composite resin has been used for the successful restoration of anterior teeth for at least the past three decades (Figures 10.1 and 10.2). There are several benefits associated with the direct use of this material for the management of TW. These include:[5]

- an opportunity to achieve an acceptable aesthetic outcome
- the option of offering a minimally invasive treatment procedure
- use as a diagnostic tool to verify acceptance of planned aesthetic and functional changes
- well tolerated by pulpal tissues
- minimally abrasive to antagonistic surfaces
- the potential for undertaking repairs and adjustments
- financial efficacy
- the option to apply restorations within a single visit.

There are also a few well-recognised disadvantages of direct resin composite restorations for the purpose of restoring patients with TW. These include:

- a relatively higher rate of wear rate (in comparison to metals and ceramics) and a possible inadequate wear resistance for use amongst posterior teeth
- a predisposition towards fracture(s), although there is evidence that direct composite restorations perform better in this respect compared with indirect restorations[6]
- a tendency to develop discolouration and staining when compared to ceramic materials
- the need for optimal moisture control, as is the case for any adhesive minimally invasive technique, especially indirect restorations
- the complexity of application, particularly in relation to the restoration of the occlusal surfaces and the inter-proximal areas, which require a skilled operator.

Direct composite resin restorations are also frequently prescribed as medium-term restorations for some cases of TW, sometimes as a prelude to the planned application of more invasive and costly conventional restorations (where there is also likely to be the need to implement macroscopically irreversible changes to the dental hard tissues). In this way, direct resin restorations can serve a *diagnostic purpose.* Their placement in a minimally invasive manner allows for ready adjustments (by addition or removal of material) to be made until all parties achieve aesthetic and functional satisfaction and adaptation (or, in the worst-case scenario, allow for some element of treatment reversal).[1]

Localised treatment for TW: Several studies have evaluated the efficacy of resin composite to treat wear of the *anterior dentition* in the short to medium term (2–6 years). The outcomes of these studies are summarised in Table 10.1. Some data for indirect resin composite restorations are also included in Table 10.1 as these restorations are placed together with directly fabricated restorations. However, the role of indirect resin restorations is discussed in further detail below.

In general, very acceptable survival rates (at or about 90%) have been described for the use of direct resin restoration to treat localised anterior TW in the short to medium term.[4,7,8] In many of the patient cases included in the studies, restorations were placed in the *supra-occlusal position*, utilising the concept of *Dahl phenomenon/relative-axial movement*, as alluded to in Chapter 5.

In the short to medium term, mechanical failure (including complete bulk fracture, marginal fracture, and chipping of material) appears to be a concern with the use of this material when placed directly for the treatment of the anterior dentition. The selection of an appropriate form of resin-based material, the thickness of the material applied, as well as the filler volume may be important factors to consider in attempting to enhance the longevity of the restoration placed. Indeed, micro-filled resin preparations are perhaps better avoided and hybrid composites preferred when managing tooth surfaces where occlusal loading is likely to be encountered, such as amongst patients where bruxist tendencies are likely to be influential in the pathogeneses of the wear pattern seen.

Whilst high success with placing restorations in supra-occlusion can be expected for patients who present with aesthetic and/or functional demands, careful patient selection is paramount. In the study by Hemmings et al.[7] the process for the re-establishment of occlusal contacts following the placement of restorations in supra-occlusion was reported to be less predictable amongst patients that presented with a gross Class III malocclusion and mandibular facial asymmetry. However, in some cases tooth movement occurred rapidly, where the element of mandibular repositioning was postulated to account for movement taking place at faster rate for such patients. Mandibular repositioning often precedes the process of dento-alevolar compensation, as discussed in Chapter 5. Adverse tooth movements such as splaying were not seen to occur in the study by Hemmings et al. either,[7] perhaps emphasising the importance of good periodontal health and alveolar bone support when planning restorative care in this manner. This observation, coupled with the general lack of biological complications associated with pulpal, periapical, periodontal and temporomandibular joint related signs/symptoms has also been reported in other studies, with the use of resin composite restorations (when also placed in the supra-occlusal position), but careful patient selection is critical.[4]

In relation to medium- to longer-term studies documenting the survival of direct localised anterior resin restorations to treat TW, the published data is somewhat more diverse.

Table 10.1 A summary of some of the studies that have been undertaken in relation to the use of resin composite to treat localised TW for the short- to medium-term restoration of worn anterior teeth.

Study	Number of patients/number of teeth/ details of note	Duration of study/ design of study	Results	Conclusions/comments
Hemmings et al.[7]	16 patients/ 104 restorations/ restorations placed at increased OVD – posterior disclusion of 1–4 mm	30 months	89% of restorations in service, mean time of 4.6 months for re-establishment of occlusal contacts (ranging from 1 to 11 months); 93/104 restorations in service	Direct composites feasible for short- to medium-term care Hybrid materials (six failures) outperformed micro-filled resins (33 failures) Good level of patient satisfaction reported
Redman et al.[8]	225 restorations placed in 31 patients; 97 direct hybrid, 37 micro-filled materials, 73 indirect ceromer ('Artglass').	5 months to 6 years	Good short- to medium-term success rate, higher probability of failure with direct materials after first 5 years; indirect materials performed well but minor wear was highlighted	Restorations placed in Class II Div 2 displayed higher probability of failure
Poyser et al.[4]	18 patients/168 restorations; randomised split mouth trial involving mandibular anterior teeth, placed 0.5 mm to 5.0 mm in supra-occlusion	2.5 years of service	6% showed complete failure; occlusal contacted re-established within a mean time of 6.2 months	No reported endodontic, periodontal or TMJ problems when placing restorations in supra occlusion High level of patient satisfaction Marginal breakdown and staining were commonly recorded

OVD, occlusal vertical dimension; TMJ, temporomandibular joint.

Whilst the outcomes of an 8-year prospective study reported a very acceptable treatment outcome with an overall failure rate of 7% amongst a sample of just over 1000 restorations,[9] data presented by other groups have been far less favourable.[10–12]

Gulamali et al.[10] reported a median survival time for 283 restorations (comprising direct and indirect restorations) at 10-year follow-up of 5.8 years, with 90% of their sample of restorations showing signs of major and minor failure due to factors such as wear, marginal discoloration, and/or fracture. Interestingly, as part of this study the survival of replaced restorations was reported to be 4.8 years, and it was postulated by the authors that further complications may be expected where there was a greater reliance on dentine bonding, indicating that TW was severe and that mechanical retention and ferrule of the restoration played a less important role. Little difference was also reported between the performance of direct and indirect restorations, although higher levels of minor failures were seen in association with indirect restorations. However, given that indirect restorations were likely chosen for more severe cases of TW, this may explain the observations reported by the authors. Higher levels of success were also reported amongst patients with Class III incisor relationships when compared to Class I or Class II Div 2. Failures in the latter category may possibly be accounted for by the higher levels of shear and tensile forces setting up stress into the restorations with such incisor relationships.[8,10]

Analogously, Bartlett and Varma[11] reported a success rate of 83%, with failures primarily due to chipping or bulk fracture; 63% of the patients included showed the presence of at least one fracture. It was suggested that operator skill and the aetiology of the condition might have an influential role on the level of success that can be expected.

As a continuation of the work published by Poyser et al.,[4] Al-Khayatt et al.[12] carried out a 7-year follow-up of 107 direct mandibular anterior restorations (placed in 15 patients). Whilst only 53% of the patients experienced survival of all the restorations, with an overall reported success rate of 51% (with no clinical problems), given that the restorations are generally amenable to repair/refurbishment (and their success rate compared favourably to the 7% success rate reported by Gulamali et al.[10]), in the view of the authors, this mode of treatment was appropriate, offering long-standing satisfactory aesthetic benefits and good long-term survival.

In summary, based on the data available, it would appear that in each of the above medium- to longer-term evaluations, the most common causes for failure with anterior resin composite restorations were de-bonding, chipping (often termed cohesive failure), bulk fracture, wear, and discolouration. In each case, biological complications were seldom encountered, reflecting the specific risk profile of the patients. The importance of appropriate posterior support was also emphasised in the study by Milosevic and Burnside.[9]

Long-term data for the use of resin composite for the management of the worn dentition is also very much lacking. One study comparing the survival of direct and indirect restorations for the treatment of advanced TW over the course of a 10-year assessment period reported a survival rate of 62.0% for all direct resin-bonded composite restorations (58.9% for anterior resin-bonded composite restorations) and 74.5% for indirect conventionally retained restorations.[13] Bulk fracture was noted as the most common mode of failure for the former, which were readily addressed conservatively by either repair or replacement. In contrast, failures of the indirect restorations were generally of a catastrophic nature, frequently involving complete loss of the restorations, which frequently necessitated subsequent endodontic treatment or a dental extraction. Interestingly, a promising survival rate of 78% was described for directly bonded resin composites placed in the anterior region.

Generalised treatment for TW: Data for the prognosis of direct resin composite restorations to manage generalised TW appears to be somewhat limited and, as for the evaluation of anterior restorations, is also variable. Bartlett and Sundaram[14] reported a poor prognosis for direct composite resin restorations when applying micro-filled based materials to restore worn posterior occluding surfaces amongst patients with parafunctional tooth grinding/clenching habits. An overall failure rate of 50% was determined over an observation period of 3 years for direct restorations. Failures amongst posterior teeth may be accounted for by the fact that material is commonly inadvertently applied to certain areas in thin sections, which may fracture, flex, crack or chip. The choice of resin (micro-filled) may also have influenced the outcomes determined.

In contrast, Schmidlin et al.[15] and Attin et al.[16] have reported a very favourable outcome for 85 direct hybrid composite resin restorations used to treat posterior segmental wear after a mean observation time of 5.5 years. In both studies, fine hybrid composite resin products were used, but marginal discolouration, marginal deterioration, and some loss of surface texture and wear should be expected. The provision of a post-operative occlusal splint should also be given due consideration.

Data from a larger study by Hamburger et al.[17] in which a full treatment of all anterior and posterior worn teeth was performed has also described a good clinical performance outcome (2.2% annual failure rate) and high levels of patient satisfaction. In this study 18 patients with generalised severe TW were treated using 332 direct composite resin restorations placed at an increased occlusal vertical dimension, in which posterior restorations were made with a highly filled hybrid composite material. The status of the restorations was evaluated after a period up to 12 years and patients were interviewed about their satisfaction with the restorative treatment using a visual analogue scale (VAS). Recently, a study of Loomans et al.[18] showed a good annual failure rate at 3.5 years of 2–3% for 34 patients with generalised severe TW. In total 1256 direct composite resin restorations were placed in increased vertical dimension. This study showed that when anterior restorations placed in increased vertical dimension were placed in two sessions instead of one session for the palatal build-up and buccal veneer, significantly more problems at the incisal interface occurred in the form of marginal ditching and fractures. This indicates that even when a repair protocol including sandblasting and the use of a silane coupling agent is applied, a restoration placed in increments in one session is significantly more resistant to failure then a restoration placed in two sessions, which relies on repair techniques in the interface.

In conclusion, there appears to be some evidence to support the effective role of direct resin restorations for at least the medium-term management of TW.

Such restorations may indeed serve a diagnostic purpose in allowing the patient to test drive the functional-aesthetic prescription, which may be substituted for alternative dental materials as discussed below at a later point in time. However, the lack of evidence for the longevity of those alternative materials, especially in the long term, for this type of patient and the disadvantage of not being able to redo a traditional build-up case in a simple way, also offers the possibility to choose for a medium long longevity of 10 years for a build-up with direct composites and redo the case for a second round in a dynamic restorative treatment concept as described by Creugers.[19]

Careful material selection, the availability of factors conducive to adhesive dentistry, and good operator skills/experience appear to be key factors. Patients must be advised of the potential regular need for polishing, repair, and occasional replacement when prescribing direct resin composites for the treatment of TW. For patients who display a tendency towards bruxism, the prescription of a post-operative occlusal splint should perhaps be given due consideration.

However, caution needs to be applied when making comparisons between studies that look at restorative success/survival due to any possible diversity in their restorative and investigatory protocols.

10.2.2 Indirect Composite Resin Restorations

The general use of indirect composite resin restorations was first described in the mid-1970s. However, only in recent times have material formulations been introduced into the marketplace that possess the desired mechanical properties and aesthetic values to provide a possible alternative to the use of dental ceramics. Most contemporary indirect composite resin products are based on hybrid resins that offer a superior level of fracture resistance (when compared to micro filled resins).

Indirect resin restorations offer some primary advantages over direct counterparts, e.g. a reduced level of polymerisation shrinkage (as this takes place extra-orally), the ability to apply further treatment after the initial curing phase, and a better polished and anatomically correct laboratory fabricated restoration.

In general, however, the advantages of indirect composite resin restorations when used in the management of cases of TW include:[5]

- improved control over occlusal contour and vertical dimension when compared to direct restorations, particularly in the case of a larger number of multiple restorations
- perhaps less time involved chairside, although this may be greatly operator dependant
- the potential to add to and repair relatively simply intra-orally (only an advantage when compared to ceramic or zirconia materials)
- aesthetically superior to cast metal restorations
- less abrasive than indirect ceramic restorations
- superior wear resistance when compared to direct materials (potentially these materials also have a higher fracture strength than direct composites, but results from Loomans et al.[6] show that indirect composite resin restoration in the posterior area demonstrates significantly more fracture than direct

composite resin restorations, which also may be due to the more complicated adhesive procedure

- polymerisation shrinkage negated intra-orally, other than at the level of the resin-luting agent.

The disadvantages include:[5]

- inferior marginal fit (versus direct, metal, and ceramic)
- restorations may be bulky
- requires at least two appointments, comparable to other indirect techniques
- laboratory costs
- may require the removal of hard tissue undercuts
- cementation line may require masking with direct materials
- it is a complex adhesive procedure in which different substrates have to be adhesively bonded (dentin, enamel, indirect composite etc.) and the possible inadequate fracture resistance for posterior use.

According to Wendt[20] the hardness and wear resistance of certain composite resins may be further enhanced by dry heating after the light-curing phase. A slow rate of heating has also been postulated to cause continued or 'extended' polymerisation, resulting in a higher degree of conversion and culminating in a greater molecular size as well as annealing of polymer chains, which has been suggested to reduce the potential for residual strain formation within the polymer matrix and a concomitantly increased ability to flex with the tissue when an occlusal load is applied (a feature which ceramics do not display and which may account for their increased level of brittleness).

An alternative to the heat treatment process includes the application of a slower rate of polymerisation (which has been suggested to improve the potential for a greater level of movement of molecular chains and thereby increase the potential for energising activation sites) and the elimination of internal porosities within the resin matrix (which may occur during conventional light curing).[21]

In relation to the *management of localised anterior TW*, further to some of the data discussed above, a very acceptable short- to medium-term success rate of 96% was reported by Gow and Hemmings.[22] In the latter study, 75 teeth displaying signs of palatal TW were restored with indirect resin composite palatal veneers (Artglass) over an observation period of 2 years; 13 cases required minor repairs, which were readily achieved intra-orally with the use of direct materials. Many of these cases were fixed Dahl appliances. Very favourable outcomes were also described by Redman et al.[8] whereby over 70 cases of localised anterior maxillary TW were treated by the application of an indirect ceromer, although a high incidence of minor wear was described as occurring on these restorations.

In relation to the medium term, Vialati et al.[23] have described very acceptable functional and aesthetic outcomes for a technique involving the use of indirect composite veneers to treat palatal surface wear, with the labial surfaces usually being restored using porcelain veneers – no complete or major failures were reported amongst a healthy sample of cases. Another comparable approach has been described combining the use of indirect and direct resin composite restorations, in which the palatal aspect of the restoration was formed indirectly and the labial portion developed directly following the cementation of the indirect palatal composite veneers.[24]

Whilst the general application of *indirect composite restorations with cuspal coverage on posterior teeth* has been reported to be very successful (amongst teeth *not* necessarily displaying signs of TW),[25] the results of a study by Bartlett and Sundaram[14] have provided less promising levels of clinical performance, where indirect cusp coverage (micro-filled) composite resin restorations were used to treat cases of posterior TW amongst patients with TW. An overall failure rate of 28% over an evaluation period of 3 years was described by the latter group; fracture and complete loss were the most common modes of failure. The authors concluded that the use of resin composites (of either direct or indirect variety) to restore worn posterior teeth should be contraindicated, but the relatively small sample size, and patient and material selection should be given due consideration.

Preliminary results from a clinical study by Loomans et al.[6] showed that for molars indirect composites showed more fractures compared to direct composites when TW patients were built-up in increased vertical dimension with adhesive restorations. Care is therefore advocated when applying indirect composites in these circumstances and particularly in bruxists.

10.3 The Use of Cast Metal (Nickel/Chromium or Type III/IV) Gold Alloys

Traditionally, conventionally retained indirect restorations fabricated from cast alloys have been used to restore worn teeth/tooth surfaces where aesthetic requirements are not of paramount importance. Smales and Berekally[13] reported a relatively good long-term prognosis for full veneer gold crown restorations used to manage worn posterior teeth, albeit for a relatively small sample size.

With the advent of chemically active resin luting cements containing agents such as 4-META or dimethacrylate (whereby phosphate ester groups are incorporated into the BisGMA resin), it has been possible to form a chemical bond between *cast adhesive restorations* and dental hard tissues with a high level of predictability. The latter has reduced the need for aggressive tooth preparations. Type III gold alloy and alloys based on nickel-chromium (Ni–Cr) are the most commonly used for the fabrication of fixed metallic adhesive restorations, such as palatal veneers or adhesive onlay restorations (Figure 10.3). The terms *gold hats* and *gold bonnets* have been used synonymously with that of posterior adhesive onlays.

Ni–Cr alloys offer improved bond strengths to resin luting agents and a higher modulus of elasticity (thereby enabling application in thinner sections), in conjunction with more conservative tooth preparation(s) than Type III gold alloys. Type III gold alloys, however, offer easier working properties and superior polish ability (because of a higher relative value of elongation and lower hardness, respectively) and superior wear characteristics and marginal fit.

The advantages of adhesive cast restorations when applied to worn occluding surfaces include the following:[5]

- they may be fabricated in thin sections (0.5 mm)
- a very accurate, predictable fit is attainable
- there is minimal wear of antagonistic surfaces
- they are protective of residual tooth structure
- they are suitable for posterior restorations amongst parafunctional patients
- they are placed supra-gingivally, therefore are conducive to good periodontal health and offer simplification of technique with regards to tooth preparation and impression making
- minimal tooth preparation required.

Disadvantages include the following:

- they may be cosmetically unacceptable due to the 'shine through' of metallic grey
- they may have very limited use amongst anterior teeth which display wear of the incisal edge
- adhesive cast restorations do not offer ease of repair intra-orally
- there is a need for copious, good-quality enamel to create an acceptable bond interface
- close proximal contacts with adjacent teeth amongst posterior teeth may pose a concern with the application of resin bonded onlay restorations[26]
- difficulty with the placement of provisional restorations
- cost, due to the increasing price of precious metal alloys.
- lack of evidence from clinical studies indicating long-term success for this type of restoration for TW patients.

In relation to the success of cast metal, adhesively retained restorations for the treatment of TW, the available data appears to be very limited. Nohl et al.[27] reported a success rate of 89% for metal palatal veneers, whereby 210 cast metal palatal veneers were prescribed and observed over a period of 56 months. The use of a chemically active resin composite luting system was shown to be more effective than the use of a glass polyalkenoate cement.

Channa et al.[28] undertook a 5-year analysis of the clinical performance of 158 gold adhesive onlays to restore posterior occlusal surfaces, many of which were prescribed for the conservative management of posterior TW. A promising survival rate of 89% was reported, with a small proportion of the restorations being placed in a supra-occlusal location. The prime cause of failure was wear of the metal alloy, which resulted in cement exposure and subsequent de-bonding.

10.4 Adhesive Ceramic Restorations

Adhesive ceramic restorations can also be used for the treatment of the aesthetic zone affected by TW. Restorations may take the form of bonded veneer restorations to ceramic crowns.

Ceramic restorations when used in the management of cases of TW have the potential to provide:[5]

- superior aesthetics (depending on where the margin is located)
- good abrasion resistance
- lower relative surface free energy compared to resin composites, thus less susceptibility to staining
- a higher level of gingival tissue tolerance.

However, such restorations are:

- brittle and prone to fracture unless applied in bulk, which may necessitate considerable tooth reduction and be associated potentially with higher failure rates amongst patients who display signs of wear by parafunctional tooth clenching and grinding habits
- potentially abrasive to the opposing dentition (particularly in the case of feldspathic porcelains); glazed porcelain has been suggested to be 40 times more abrasive to antagonistic surfaces than Type III gold[29]
- difficult to repair intra-orally
- difficult to adjust
- susceptible to degradation wear in acidic environments
- costly.

It has been suggested that the delamination risk of ceramics is high amongst posterior teeth where there may be signs of severe TW associated with bruxist tendencies.[30] Data for the use of adhesive ceramic restorations to treat TW is often limited to the availability of case reports.[31,32]

Walls[33] described the successful application of *porcelain veneers* for the treatment of wear, but the sample size was relatively small (fewer than 60 restorations). Whilst bulk fracture and marginal staining/discolouration were described, with the contemporary advances in adhesive dentistry and ceramic technology that have taken place over the past two decades, differing outcomes may be expected.

In relation to the prescription of *all-ceramic crowns*, Milosevic[34] reported a relatively low failure rate of 15.5% of over a median follow-up period of 72 months amongst a sample of 161 zirconia crowns used to restore severe anterior TW. Failures were attributable to total de-bond or to minor delamination chips within the ceramic layer. The presence of an edge-to-edge incisor relationship, as well as an underlying tendency towards developing TW because of attrition or bruxism, was also linked to a higher risk of failure.

A factor to account for the lack of data concerning the use of adhesive ceramics as the initial choice for the treatment of severe wear may be the increased treatment cost that can be associated with the use of adhesive ceramic restorations, especially given the knowledge that some patients may fail to accept/adapt to the functional and/or aesthetic rehabilitation provided. The use of adhesive ceramics may, however, be considered suitable amongst cases that may have been successfully stabilised using direct resin composites, as described by Magne et al.[35] Given the propensity of ceramics towards delamination and chipping, it has been suggested that an occlusal splint should be provided for nocturnal use (post-restoration placement) for all wear cases treated with ceramics to protect restorations from parafunctional habits which may be associated with premature degradation.[36]

With advances in digital dentistry, CAD/CAM manufactured restorations using high-density polymeric materials may permit the use of more robust materials that may be applied in thinner sections than dental ceramic, as described by a set of case reports presented by Edelhoff et al.[37]

10.5 Summary

The successful management of a patient presenting with signs of pathological TW is dependent on the clinician having a good knowledge of and ability to apply the principles of occlusion, and the available materials and techniques for restoring such cases with a high level of predictability. Patients with a bruxist habit are a high-risk group as are cases where considerable coronal tooth tissue has been lost. Patients with TW form a distinct group and extrapolation of the survival and longevity results from evidence collected from restorations placed in patients without TW to this group should be viewed with caution.

The importance of informed consent and contingency planning when providing complex restorative care cannot be over-emphasised. This requires an effective working knowledge of the materials available to the dental practitioner.

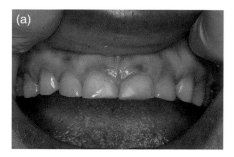 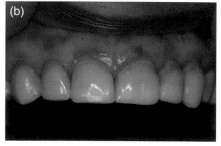

Figure 10.1 (a) Patient with TW. (b) Patient shown in (a) with anterior worn teeth restored with direct composite.

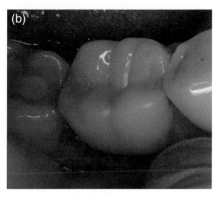
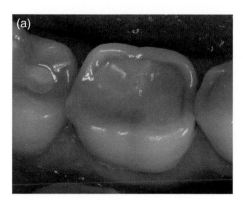

Figure 10.2 (a) Patient with a worn and sensitive lower right first molar tooth. (b) The lower right first molar tooth as shown in (a) has been restored with direct composite and this view was taken at a recall appointment.

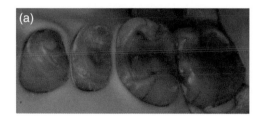
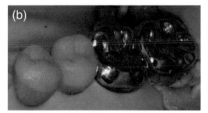

Figure 10.3 (a) Patient with TW. (b) Patient shown in (a) with the premolars restored with lithium disilicate and molars restored with gold alloy onlays immediately after cementation.

References

1 Mehta, S.B., Banerji, S., Millar, B.J., and Saures-Fieto, J.M. (2012). Current concepts in tooth wear management. Part 4. An overview of the restorative techniques and materials commonly applied for the management of tooth wear. *Br. Dent. J.* 212 (4): 169–177.

2 Mesko, M., Sarkis-Onofre, R., Cenci, M. et al. (2016). Rehabilitation of severely worn teeth. A systematic review. *J. Dent.* 48: 9–15.

3 Loomans, B., Opdam, N., Attin, T. et al. (2017). Severe tooth wear: European consensus statement on management guidelines. *J. Adhes. Dent.* 19: 111–119.

4 Poyser, N., Porter, R., Briggs, P., and Kelleher, M. (2007). Demolition experts: management of the parafunctional patient 2: restorative management strategies. *Dent. Update* 34: 262–268.

5 Kilpatrick, N. and Mahoney, E. (2004). Dental erosion: Part 2. The management of dental erosion. *N. Z. Dent. J.* 2: 42–47.

6 Loomans, B.A.C., Bougatsias, L., Sterenborg, B.A.M.M. et al. (2018). Survival of direct and indirect composites restorations in toothwear patients. *IADR*, Abstract #0338. Poster at the IADR Conference 2018 (Publication pending).

7 Hemmings, K., Darbar, U., and Vaughan, S. (2000). Tooth wear treated with direct composite at an increased vertical dimension; results at 30 months. *J. Prosthet. Dent.* 83: 287–293.

8 Redman, C., Hemmings, K., and Good, J. (2003). The survival and clinical performance of resin based composite restorations used to treat localised anterior tooth wear. *Br. Dent. J.* 194: 566–572.

9 Milosevic, A. and Burnside, G. (2016). The survival of direct composite restorations in the management of severe tooth wear including attrition and erosion: a prospective 8-year study. *J. Dent.* 44: 13–19.

10 Gulamali, A., Hemmings, K., Tredwin, C., and Petrie, A. (2011). Survival analysis of composite Dahl restorations provided to manage localised anterior tooth wear (ten year follow-up). *Br. Dent. J.* 211: E9.

11 Bartlett, D. and Varma, S. (2017). A retrospective audit of the outcome of composites used to restore worn teeth. *Br. Dent. J.* 223: 33–36.

12 Al-Khayatt, A., Ray-Chaudhuri, A., Poyser, N. et al. (2013). Direct composite restorations for the worn mandibular anterior dentition: a 7-year follow up of a prospective randomised controlled split-mouth clinical trial. *J. Oral Rehabil.* 40: 389–401.

13 Smales, R. and Berekally, T. (2007). Long term survival of direct and indirect restorations placed for the treatment of advanced tooth wear. *Eur. J. Prosthodont. Restor. Dent.* 15: 2–6.

14 Bartlett, D. and Sundaram, G. (2006). An up to 3-year randomized clinical study comparing indirect and direct resin composites used to restore worn posterior teeth. *Int. J. Prosthodont.* 19 (6): 613–617.

15 Schmidlin, P., Filli, T., Imfeld, C. et al. (2009). Three tear evaluation of posterior vertical bite reconstruction using direct resin composite – a case series. *Oper. Dent.* 34: 102–108.

16 Attin, T., Filli, T., Imfeld, C., and Schmidlin, P. (2012). Composite vertical bite reconstructions in eroded dentitions after 5.5 years: case series. *J. Oral Rehabil.* 39: 73–79.

17 Hamburger, J., Opdam, N., Bronkhorst, E. et al. (2011). Clinical performance of direct composite restorations for treatment of severe tooth wear. *J. Adhes. Dent.* 13: 585–593.

18 Loomans, B.A.C., Kreulen, C.M., Huijs-Visser, H.E.C.E. et al. (2018). Clinical performance of full rehabilitations with direct composite in severe tooth wear patients: 3.5 years results. *J. Dent.* 70: 97–103. https://doi.org/10.1016/j.jdent.2018.01.001. Epub 2018 Jan 12. PubMed PMID:29339203.

19 Creugers, N.H. (2003). Minimal invasive dentistry. A revolutionary concept? *Ned. Tijdschr. Tandheelkd.* 110: 215–217. Article in Dutch.

20 Wendt, S.L. (1987). The effect of heat used as a secondary cure upon the physical properties of three composite resins. Dimetral tensile strength, compressive strength and marginal dimensional stability. *Quintessence Int.* 18 (4): 265–271.

21 Wendt, S.L. and Leinfelder, K.F. (1992). Clinical evaluation of a heat treated resin composite inlay. 3 year results. *Am. J. Dent.* 5: 258–262.

22 Gow, A. and Hemmings, K. (2002). The treatments of localised anterior tooth wear with indirect Artglass restorations at an increased occlusal vertical dimension. Results after 2 years. *Eur. J. Prosthodont. Restor. Dent.* 10: 101–105.

23 Vailati, F., Gruetter, L., and Belser, U. (2013). Adhesively restored anterior maxillary dentitions affected by severe erosion: up to 6-year results of a prospective clinical study. *Eur. J. Esthet. Dent.* 8 (4): 506–530.

24 Satterthwaite, J. (2012). Tooth surface loss: tools and tips for management. *Dent. Update* 39: 86–96.

25 Delipieri, S. and Bardwell, D. (2006). Clinical evaluation of direct cuspal coverage with posterior composite resin restorations. *J. Esthet. Restor. Dent.* 18: 256–267.

26 Yap, A. (1995). Cuspal coverage with resin bonded metal onlays. *Dent. Update*: 403–406.

27 Nohl, F., King, P., Harley, K., and Ibbetson, R. (1997). Retrospective survey of resin retained cast metal palatal veneers for treatment of anterior palatal tooth wear. *Quintessence Int.* 28: 7–14.

28 Chana, H., Kelleher, M., Briggs, P., and Hooper, R. (2000). Clinical evaluation of resin bonded gold alloy veneers. *J. Prosthet. Dent.* 83: 294–300.

29 Wada, T. (1986). Development of a new adhesive material and its properties. In: *Proceedings of the international symposium on adhesive Prosthodontics* (eds. L. Gettleman, M.M.A. Vrijhoef, Y. Uchiyama), 9–19.

30 Dorri, M. (2013). All ceramic toot-supported single crowns have acceptable 5-year survival rates. *Evid. Based Dent.* 14: 47.

31 Malkoc, M., SEvimay, M., and Yaprak, E. (2009). The use of zirconium and feldspathic porcelain in the management of the severely worn dentition: a case report. *Eur. J. Dent.* 3: 75–80.

32 Nam, J. and Tokutomi, H. (2015). Using zirconia-based prosthesis in complete-mouth reconstruction treatment for worn dentition with altered vertical dimension of occlusion. *Prosthet. Dent.* 113: 81–85.

33 Walls, A. (1995). The use of adhesively retained all-porcelain veneers during the management of fractured and worn anterior teeth. Part 2. Clinical results after 5 years of follow up. *Br. Dent. J.* 178: 337–340.

34 Milosevic, A. (2014). The survival of zirconia based crowns (Lava) in the management of severe anterior tooth wear up to 7-years follow-up. *Oral Biol. Dent.* 2: 1–7.

35 Magne, P., Magne, M., and Bleser, U. (2007). Adhesive restorations, centric relation, and the Dahl principal: minimally invasive approaches to localised anterior tooth erosion. *Eur. J. Esthet. Dent.* 2: 260–273.

36 Oh, W., DeLong, R., and Anusavice, K. (2002). Factors affecting enamel and ceramic wear: a literature review. *J. Prosthet. Dent.* 87: 451–459.

37 Edelhoff, D., Beuer, F., Schweiger, J. et al. (2012). CAD/CAM-generated high-density polymer restorations for the pre-treatment of complex cases: a case report. *Quintessence Int.* 43: 457–467.

Further Reading

Briggs, P., Djemal, S., Chana, H., and Kelleher, M. (1998). Young adult patients with established dental erosion – what should be done? *Dent. Update* 25: 166–170.

Bartlett, D. (2016). A personal perspective and update on erosive tooth wear – 10 years on: Part 2. Restorative management. *Br. Dent. J.* 221: 167–171.

11

The Principles and Clinical Management of Localised Anterior Tooth Wear

11.1 Introduction

In Chapter 4, the subdivision of wear cases as being localised or generalised was alluded to. The latter classification can prove to be of benefit when attempting to plan care, which can often be a complex process. Success when undertaking restorative rehabilitation for tooth wear (TW) is to a large extent dependent on meticulous treatment planning, as well as the effective technical execution of the treatment stages. The aim of this chapter is to consider the latter in relation to the clinical management of *localised anterior TW*.

11.1.1 Planning Considerations

According to Mehta et al.[1] there several factors to consider when planning the restorative rehabilitation of localised anterior TW. These include:

1) The pattern of anterior tooth surface loss
2) The inter-occlusal space availability
3) The space requirements of the dental restorations being proposed
4) The quantity and quality of available dental hard tissue and enamel, respectively
5) The aesthetic demands of the patient.

In relation to the *pattern of anterior maxillary TW*, Chu et al.[2] have described three categories:

1) TW that is limited to the palatal surfaces only
2) TW involving the palatal and incisal edges, with reduced clinical crown height
3) TW limited to labial surfaces only.

Given the impact of prescribing restorative materials that are of low aesthetic value, for cases involving visible surfaces (as with the former two categories) it is most likely that restorative techniques will involve the use of tooth-coloured aesthetic materials (at least on visible surfaces). Consequently, metallic restorations, such as metal palatal veneers, have limited use in these cases. In contrast, for

Practical Procedures in the Management of Tooth Wear, First Edition. Subir Banerji, Shamir Mehta, Niek Opdam and Bas Loomans.
© 2020 John Wiley & Sons Ltd. Published 2020 by John Wiley & Sons Ltd.
Companion website: www.wiley.com/go/banerji/toothwear

cases where the pathology is palatal only, metal palatal veneers may prove to be an appropriate restorative option.

11.2 Inter-occlusal space availability[1]

For most patients, the wearing away of the dental hard tissues is accompanied by the process of dento-alveolar compensation (as discussed in Chapter 6). This physiological compensatory mechanism allows occlusal contacts to be maintained. However, the ensuing loss of inter-occlusal space poses a major conundrum for the restorative dentist.

In some cases (particularly where the rate of TW may be very rapid, or compensatory mechanisms evolve at a relatively slower rate, or in the case of a patient with an anterior open bite, deep overbite or increased overjet) an adequate space/inter-occlusal may be available between the *upper and lower dentition in centric occlusion (CO)/the inter-cuspal position (ICP)* that may be utilised to accommodate dental restorations without the concomitant need to either reduce healthy tooth tissue or follow a reorganised approach. Under such circumstances, adhesively retained restorations may simply be bonded into the available space to restore form, aesthetics, and function.

For most of cases of TW, however, adequate inter-occlusal clearance is not available. Under such circumstances, traditional prosthodontic protocols have usually involved the need to create space to accommodate conventionally retained restorations by carrying out further tooth reduction (sometimes also requiring the need for pre-restorative periodontal surgery). The risks of adopting this approach are discussed at length in Chapter 10.

In some cases, further space may be gained in order to accommodate the required inter-occlusal clearance by adopting a *reorganised approach*, whereby the presence of any slides (vertical and/or horizontal) between the ICP and the first centric relation contact position (CRCP) may reduce, or in some cases negate, the requirement to carry out further tooth reduction to provide restorative care at a physiological occlusal vertical dimension. The feasibility of the latter approach (as discussed in Chapter 6) is perhaps best confirmed by accurate study casts mounted in centric relation on a semi-adjustable (or fully adjustable) articulator.

Occasionally, the space created by such a reorganised approach may be sufficient to permit the use of more rigid materials such as metallic alloys that require less bulk thickness to ensure longevity, but not enough for the use of more elastic materials such as resin composite. However, sometimes the plan to undertake a reorganised approach for the rehabilitation of localised anterior wear may culminate in several teeth (often unaffected teeth) needing restorations to maintain occlusal stability, which will, of course, further compound the complexity of care, the maintenance requirements, and procedural fees.

Under circumstances, when localised TW is present on anterior teeth, whilst the amount of wear in the posterior areas does not justify placing multiple restorations in increased vertical dimension of occlusion (VDO), the placement of restorations to treat localised wear in the supra-occlusal position utilising the concepts of the *Dahl concept/relative axial movement* (as discussed in Chapter 6) may be given due consideration.

It has been suggested that where a patient is to be treated by the means of a fixed Dahl appliance/restoration, they must be advised of the (limited) risks of initial post-operative discomfort, problems of food collection on posterior occlusal surfaces, and possible difficulties associated with the eating of certain types of food such as lettuce and ham, as discussed further below. However, in the experience of the authors, most patients adapt well to the absence of posterior occlusal contacts within a few weeks. Another risk which the patient should be made aware of is that the posterior teeth do not re-establish contact and occlusion, and as a result may require further posterior restorative treatment. Following a partial build-up of the occlusion in the anterior teeth, the occlusal scheme should also be reviewed periodically post-operatively at intervals between 3 and 12 months, depending on the case.[3]

The *space requirements of the restorations* is also a key considerations. This will be determined by the minimal thickness a dental material can be applied to the affected surface to provide resilient and predictable function

The *quantity and quality of remaining dental hard tissue* will have an obvious impact, as discussed in Chapter 10. In extreme cases of anterior maxillary, the only remaining options may be to consider the use of an overdenture or overlay denture, conventional denture or dental implants.

The *aesthetic requirements of the patient* are also important to consider. The use of metal palatal veneers may impart a dulled appearance to the restored tooth and sometimes the visible display of metal on incisal edges.[1] It is also often very difficult to consistently gain superior aesthetic outcomes using resin composite, even with the use of layering techniques; such materials may discolour, wear, and chip away, whilst the application of conventional porcelain fused to metal restorations may result in visible 'black margins', especially when used in conjunction with surgical crown lengthening procedures, culminating in unaesthetic and excessive black triangular spaces.

In summary, there are several key factors to consider when planning the restoration of a worn anterior maxillary dentition. It is paramount that valid informed consent is attained (supported with an appropriate written dental treatment plan), ensuring that the reasonable treatment options have been appraised in a clear, accurate, logical, balanced, and comprehensive manner. Suitable dental records should be made of any discussions that take place.

11.3 Restoration of Localised Anterior TW

Having carried out all the necessary assessments and evaluations (inclusive of occlusal and aesthetic zone appraisal) with the aid of suitably mounted accurate dental casts, decided upon the treatment approach, selected the appropriate materials/restorations, carried out an intra-oral mock up (as described in Chapter 8), and attained patient consent, the next stage in treatment provision usually involves the applying of the information collected (e.g. the wax-up) to treat the worn dentition.

As discussed in Chapter 10, a variety of dental materials may be used to restore the worn dentition. Below the technical execution of the effective transference of the determined functional-aesthetic prescription using these materials is described. Emphasis has been placed on the use of direct resin restorations, largely due to the increasingly recognised merits for the use of this material and technique for the restoration of the worn anterior dentition.

11.3.1   Direct Resin Composite

When prescribing the use of direct resin composite to treat a worn dentition, it is generally accepted that for areas of high loading, it should be applied at a minimal thickness of 1.0 mm to avoid premature failure.[4,5] Particularly within this high-risk patient group (e.g. bruxist), sufficient thickness of the restoration will provide more strength, whilst the expected wear of the composite will take longer to result in new exposure of the tooth surface. It is also important that patients are properly advised about the expected longevity of restorations, which will usually be between 5 and 10 years. Burke[6] describes a patient information leaflet that may be used in helping to advise patients about matters such as:

- difficulty with chewing for 3–6 months (especially when restorations are placed in supra-occlusion), with the need to cut up food into small pieces to avoid intestinal symptoms
- a change in tooth morphology, which may initially cause lisping
- the feeling of some tenderness on biting in the front teeth for a few days post-operative
- feeling of the bite being 'unusual' for a few days
- the lack of need for local anaesthesia and any marked tooth reduction
- the possibility that existing crowns, bridges or dentures in the posterior segments may need replacement in the future
- the expected good reliability of the restorations, although there may be a chance of debonding, staining at the margins and occasional chipping, for which longer term/ongoing care will likely be required.

A number of different direct resin composite restorative placement techniques for the restoration of the worn anterior dentition have been described in the literature, including:[7]

- total freehand application of resin composite
- combined freehand application with the direct shaping by occlusion (DSO) technique where occlusal contact is shaped by biting on a polyvinylsiloxane (PVS) stop that is made on the castings[8]
- the use of a customised PVS matrix
- the use of a customised vacuum-formed matrix (including the injection moulding technique).

Whilst the application of direct composite resin *freehand* has the potential to offer excellent aesthetic results, with the concomitant merit of restorations being placed within a single visit (without the need for taking impressions), this method of material application is considerably dependent on operator skill. The technique for undertaking freehand resin additions is summarised below.

- Select the most appropriate shade(s) of resin composite. This is best done whilst the teeth are hydrated. The use of a trial shade or a mock-up may prove beneficial.
- Hybrid materials are perhaps best used, especially on the palatal side where high forces will be encountered. A highly filled composite material has proven its suitability in the mid-term.[9,10] No clinical data on build-ups with nano-composites are available yet, and it is expected that these materials may provide less fracture resistance (due to their lower particle size) but increased wear resistance (due to the smooth surface). For the labial surfaces, the aesthetical demands are higher and a mini-filled hybrid composite or a nano-filled composite will probably be the best choice.
- It is sometimes helpful to take an appropriate colour photograph of the affected teeth/tooth. The image may be adjusted by a reduction in the contrast, which will provide a 'map' showing the chromatic variations present. This may be mimicked restoratively by using a combination of suitable shades and resin tints to enhance the aesthetic appearance of the restorations. Indeed, it is sometimes worthwhile producing a sketch of desired the post-operative outcome, including the topography of the incisal edge, which may (or may not, depending on the age of the patient) have considerable character such as stains and the presence of well-demarcated mamelons.
- In relation to the management of a worn maxillary anterior dentition (given that it is generally accepted that the width of a maxillary central incisor should be approximately 1.2 times greater than its width), the use of a set of callipers to measure the width of the central incisor teeth can provide a helpful guide in determining a suitable post-operative length of these teeth as well as establishing equal width of the central incisors.
- Provide an appropriate form of isolation. When possible the use of a rubber dam is recommended, although for certain techniques this might be impossible. In such situations, a combination of an Optragate device (Ivoclar Vivadent), cotton rolls, and suction can be used.
- Having managed any defective pre-existing restorations, some operators may elect to initially prepare a bevel at the facial enamel surface and prepare the palatal enamel to receive a butt finish. The latter may help to improve micro-mechanical retention as well as the aesthetic outcome. Some authors also advocate the use of a double bevel on the facial surface, a more coronal bevel at a width of 1 mm placed at 45° to the long axis of the tooth (to which the dentine shade is matched), and a more diffuse bevel, placed apically to the first bevel, 2–3 mm in width at approximately 20° to the long axis. The use of a rugby ball-shaped bur may be helpful, whilst the application of a brown silicone rubber point can help to remove any unsupported enamel.
- Having thoroughly cleaned the teeth using oil-free pumice slurry or air-abrasion, in cases where an increase in the occlusal vertical dimension (OVD) is not being planned the centric stops should be marked up using articulating paper.

- The adjacent teeth should be separated using a suitable form of matrix. This can be achieved by the placement of a suitable matrix, such as cellulose acetate strip(s), a metal matrix or polytetrafluoroethylene (PTFE) tape, depending on operator preference.
- Having prepared the tooth surface for adhesive bonding, a chosen inter-proximal matrix should be placed to encompass each of the inter-proximal areas. For this purpose, the use of a Teflon-coated *dead soft matrix* may prove particularly helpful. The matrix can be held in situ using a suitable form of dental wedge.
- The selected enamel shade should then be placed onto the affected tooth against the matrix, using the index finger of the left hand (for a right-handed operator) to support the matrix. With the use of an appropriate plastic instrument, the resin restorative material should be carefully adapted to form the palatal enamel, commonly referred to as the *palatal shelf*. A paddle-shaped instrument or an inter-proximal carver can be helpful at this stage. For severe TW cases, where the palatal surface needs sufficient bulk of material, the restorative material can be applied in bulk using the DSO technique (see Chapter 12).
- The shelf should be prepared such that it remains slightly longer than the anticipated final vertical height of the tooth. This permits subtraction during the finishing and polishing phase. The shelf should also be finished such that at this stage it is short of the inter-proximal areas. The unset resin should be cured following the manufacturer's instructions.
- The next stage involves the development of the *inter-proximal pillars*. The required shade of resin should be dispensed into one of the inter-proximal areas and with the aid of a suitable instrument (such as a burnisher) material should be adapted between the matrix and the palatal shelf. The use of a goats-hair brush can also be useful at this stage (particularly when using pre-warmed resin composite). The pillar should be built to the profile of the facial enamel layer.
- The matrix strip should next be carefully rotated over on the facial surface and the material light-cured. This process is then repeated for the fabrication of the opposing wall and the result should yield an 'envelope'.
- A dentine shade (if required) can be placed in the envelope to replace lost dentine tissue. Material should be placed to the level of the first bevel.
- With the aid of a fine-bladed instrument, the dentine layer should be finished in accordance with the desired incisal edge anatomy. Thus, for a younger patient, the dentine layer should end at a position in the envelope that is short enough to help develop the desired level of incisal edge translucency. Mamelons may also be sculpted if required and the materials light-cured. For further refinement, subsurface resin tints may be applied to the dentine layer and light-cured.
- Finally, the enamel shade is placed over the dentine layer up to the second bevel, sculpted to form the desired *emergence profile*, and subsequently cured. Some operators choose to add a final layer of translucent resin shade to enhance the aesthetics.

- The same process is repeated for the other anterior maxillary teeth. Some operators prefer the restoration of alternative teeth, which can help with the management of the inter-proximal surfaces.
- Articulating paper should be used to initially verify the desired occlusal scheme and adjustments made using a diamond bur.
- An effort should be made to assess the proportion, size, and symmetry of the restorations across the midline. Features to note are the *height to width ratio*, which should be approximately 1.2:1 for a maxillary central incisor, the relationship of the *incsal edge to the lip line and the naso-labial angle at rest*, the *placement of contact areas, embarasure spaces and connectors* in desirable positions as discussed in Chapter 4, *the axial inclination* of the restored teeth, the *morphology of the restored teeth in frontal and lateral planes,* the presence of *symmetry across the midline*, and *the overall shape of the teeth*, features that may indeed reflect upon the personality and/or facial profile of the patient. The equal width of the central incisors should be determined with a calliper.
- The use of a pencil to mark up adjustments may prove helpful.
- Adjustments can be made carefully using a needle shaped diamond bur or, where necessary, further resin added.
- *Gross finishing* may be undertaken using a set of tungsten carbide composite finishing burs, followed by the use of dental stones, such as Durastone (Shofu Dental, Japan). Prior to discharging the patient, an effort should be made to reassess the occlusion and to ensure the desired occlusal scheme.
- It is good practice to complete the polishing stage at a subsequent visit. During this visit, together with a review, *micro-characterisation of* the restorations may be performed to further enhance the aesthetic outcome.
- Finally, a layer of glycerine is applied to the restoration and light-cured to ensure polymerisation of the surface layer, which may otherwise remain unpolymerised due to the *air inhibition phenomenon.*
- A silicone key may be constructed and kept with the patient's records to guide future additions or repairs and to monitor the wear pattern of the restoration.

Where there is a need to increase the occlusal vertical dimension or place restorations in supra-occlusion, there are more techniques for doing this. One method includes starting the procedure with the *maxillary canine tooth* (assuming this requires restoration). Resin is added to determine the presence of a canine-guided occlusion, coupled with adequate inter-occlusal clearance to restore the residual anterior maxillary dentition. Once the canine teeth have been restored, the remaining teeth may be attended to, with the aim of provided canine-guided occlusion and evenly shared contacts during protrusion, verified using articulating paper. The anatomy and location of the canine teeth, commonly with a lengthy, bulbous root, renders them suitable for the process of providing posterior disclusion, as discussed in Chapter 5.

This technique is also often utilised when fabricating *canine-rise restorations* and is explained further in Chapter 12.

The DSO technique is also described in the accompanying video for this book and involves using silicon stops fabricated on the mounted casting (www.wiley.com/go/banerji/toothwear).[8] These silicon stops, which are made in the posterior areas, can be transferred to the mouth and enable patients to bite in the new OVD on the stops. In order to establish occlusion, a palatal metal matrix is placed and adjusted so that it does not interfere with the antagonist when the patient bites onto the stops. Subsequently, composite is injected at the palatal surface and shaped with hand instruments. Antagonistic teeth should be separated using petroleum jelly or Teflon tape and the patient asked to close into the stops, after which the material is polymerised. When necessary, a buccal veneer restoration can be made with direct composite. With this technique, it is recommended to start with the upper central incisors, then the lateral incisors and finally the canines. Using the DSO technique canine guidance will be obtained when suitable overbite is present. The reader is referred to the accompanying video for more details of this technique (www.wiley.com/go/banerji/toothwear).

For more challenging anterior TW cases, there is a need for a protocol that provides the operator with a greater level of control and predictability, and which offers contingency planning. This can be accomplished by the use of a *diagnostic wax-up*, which should be carefully formulated on the basis of an accurate occlusal and aesthetic prescription, as discussed in Chapter 8. The latter may be directly indexed using either a stable and firm PVS material or a stone duplicate, which can then be used to form a vacuum-formed thermoplastic template to assist with resin composite placement. Alternatively, the DSO technique is suitable for extensive cases.

Cases of anterior TW that may benefit from the use of a more controlled approach include:

- where there may be extensive TW, extending to include a significant portion of the proximal walls
- occlusal changes that may involve an overall increase in the OVD, especially where multiple posterior restorations are being planned
- where attainment of the functional or aesthetic end point may be challenging
- where is a need to apply resin composite in a 'layered' manner.

Given that it is important to ensure a preferable minimal thickness of 1.0–1.5 mm of material in all areas of functional loading, the wax patterns should be made to conform to this dimension. The occlusal end point should aim to provide even contacts in the inter-cuspal position, shared occlusal contacts upon mandibular protrusion, and a canine-guided occlusal scheme.[1,7] It should be noted that in cases where there is also TW on the posterior teeth, then this would also need to be addressed. Where TW is localised in the maxillary anterior dentition, the passive axial re-establishment of the posterior teeth following anterior build-up would allow the desired occlusal contacts to be established and this should be confirmed. There may, however, be a need to include alterations on this generic approach given the individual circumstances, such as the presence of a large direct restoration or endodotically treated tooth (particularly in the presence of a post-retained core).

The technique for the use of a polyvinylsilicone index is summarised in Table 11.1.

Table 11.1 Suggested technique for the use of a polyvinylsiloxans (PVS) index to undertake restorative rehabilitation with direct resin composite.

- Carefully inspect the diagnostic wax-up when returned from the dental laboratory. The use of a Golden Mean Gauge to ascertain the desired proportions may be helpful.
- Prepare a *palatal silicone index*, commonly referred to as a *silicone key*. The index will assist with resin placement in an incremental, layered manner and will allow the worn-down tooth to be reconstructed in an anatomical way and also optimise resin polymerisation by applying suitable increment sizes that will permit complete polymerisation. The silicone key will in essence provide a 'negative' of the occlusal prescription as established by the wax-up, allowing the occlusal prescription to be copied.
- When constructing an index, the use of a non-perforated impression tray is advised to enable the index to be separated without damaging the diagnostic wax-up, or the placement of a separator film advocated to allow for the ease of removal of the set material.
- To prepare the index, on a suitably damp dental cast of the wax-up apply the chosen PVS material. Duplication of the wax-up in stone can lead to the loss of fine detail. The use of a transparent PVS material (such as Memosil 2, Heraus Kulzer, Germany) can be helpful in permitting light-curing from a palatal direction. This is particularly relevant for cases of TW where there has been significant loss of palatal enamel, with a minimal loss of incisal edge tissue. Otherwise a putty consistency can be used.
- The PVS material should be extended to the premolar areas and wrapped around these teeth to provide support and stability. The index material should be sufficiently bulky to provide rigidity so that it does not readily exhibit flexion upon intra-oral insertion and seating. On the facial aspect, the index should only extend up to the incisal edge. Any excess material should be carefully cut away using a putty knife or a scalpel.
- Select the appropriate shade(s) of resin composite. It is worthwhile producing a hand-drawn sketch of desired the post-operative outcome, including the topography of the incisal edge.
- With an appropriate form of isolation in situ (having managed any defective pre-existing restorations), the option may be taken to initially bevel the facial enamel and prepare the palatal enamel to receive a butt finish. The latter may help to improve micro-mechanical retention as well as the aesthetic outcome.
- Thoroughly clean the teeth using oil-free pumice slurry or air abrasion. Adjacent teeth should be protected using an appropriate form of matrix as described above.
- Commence the build-up procedure on a maxillary canine tooth. Condition the surface for adhesive bonding.
- Prior to index placement, place an appropriate quantity of enamel shade on the surface of the tooth to be restored; the use of pre-warmed resin composite may prove helpful. The amount of resin dispensed will depend on the level and pattern of TW present.
- Position the index, making sure that it is correctly seated. Using the chosen instrument (a paddle-shaped instrument or an inter-proximal carver are useful for this purpose), form the *palatal enamel wall*. The use of flowable resin composites is not recommended as they will not offer the required mechanical strength.
- Place a suitable matrix to encompass both of the inter-proximal areas, commonly referred to as the *inter-proximal pillars*. The use of a Teflon-coated *dead soft matrix* may be particularly helpful as it can be shaped with a burnisher in a customised manner and will retain its form. The presence of the Teflon coating will help to prevent adhesion of the resin-based materials to the matrix. The matrix may be held in situ using a suitable form of inter-proximal wedge.

(Continued)

Table 11.1 (Continued)

- Place the selected enamel shade onto the affected tooth against the matrix strip on either the mesial or distal surface. Using the index finger of the left hand (for a right-handed operator) carefully support the matrix. Using a suitable instrument, carefully adapt the material between the matrix and the palatal shelf; the pillar should form a substitute for the enamel tissue lost in this area of the tooth.
- A goats-hair brush can be useful in adapting the material, particularly when using warmed resin composite.
- Some clinicians choose to gently 'tug' the matrix in a palatal direction to improve adaptation. The pillar should be built to the profile of the facial enamel layer.
- Carefully roll the matrix strip over on the facial surface and light-cure it. Repeat the process for the opposing wall.
- Having formed an *envelope*, apply the chosen dentine shade (if required) to replace lost dentine tissue, as described for the freehand technique above.
- Using a fine-bladed instrument, finish the dentine layer in accordance with the desired incisal edge anatomy. For a younger patient, in order to develop a translucent finish, the dentine layer should be short enough against the palatal shelf to develop the desired level of incisal edge translucency. Mamelons may also be sculpted if required using either a fine-bladed instrument or a pointed cone-shaped burnisher. Light cure the layers of composite. For further refinement, subsurface resin tints may be carefully applied to the dentine layer and light-cured.
- Finally, apply the enamel shade over the dentine layer to the second bevel and light-cure, as described above.
- The process should be repeated on the antagonistic maxillary canine tooth, followed by the restoration of the maxillary central incisor teeth and finally the lateral incisors (when restoration of the anterior maxillary segment is indicated). A similar process can be used for the mandibular dentition.
- Finish and polish accordingly.

With the advent of clear or *transparent silicones*, such as Memosil (Heraeus Kulzer, Newbury, Bucks, UK), it is possible to ensure that adequate quantities of material are applied to worn palatal surfaces (without the inclusion of major voids) and subsequently light-cured (through the matrix), which is an obvious drawback associated with the use of non-transparent materials. The lack of rigidity offered by available transparent silicones can make the accurate positioning of such indices difficult, which may culminate in the need for copious adjustments. Furthermore, the removal of 'flash' from the material may prove challenging (by its transparent nature), which will also increase the need for further alteration of the resin composite restorations post light-curing. For further details on how to fabricate and apply a PVS matrix guide, refer to Nixon et al.[11]

The use of a ***vacuum-formed matrix guide*** has been described by Daoudi and Radford.[12] They suggest that a duplicate cast poured in dental stone is formed from a diagnostic wax-up, and a vacuum-formed transparent matrix is formed in a material of choice. Mizrahi[13] has advocated that the matrix should be formed from a rigid material (to permit accurate seating) and be of approximately 1 mm in thickness. The matrix should be extended over sound teeth that do not require restoration to provide positioning stops for the matrix to remain in place when resin is applied. Small relief holes can be cut into the matrix to avoid air entrapment.

To avoid bonding of resin material to interproximal surfaces, Daoudi and Radford[17] described the interproximal placement of wedge-shaped cellulose acetate strips of approximately 4mm in length retained by means of customised wedges trimmed so that they do not interfere with the placement of the matrix. Resin is applied to the matrix (following the appropriate conditioning of the affected teeth for the purposes of adhesive bonding), firmly placed, and resin light-cured.

However, the management of interproximal excess and the inability to apply resin incrementally or indeed in layers are obvious drawbacks with this approach. Other commonly encountered problems with the use of a vacuum-formed guide include:

- difficulty with the augmentation of the interproximal areas, with gross interproximal excess being encountered
- difficulty with resin layering, resulting in monochromatic restorations, with risks of inadequate polymerisation due to incomplete light transmission to the basal layers of the material
- air entrapment
- difficulty estimating the amount of material required, often resulting in underfilling and the subsequent development of voids or gross excess, necessitating lengthy and cumbersome refinement.

The use of this method has been suggested to be unsuitable in cases of advanced severe TW.[12] To overcome the problem of interproximal excess, the use of a technique that involves the restoration of alternative teeth to permit the complete establishment of individual tooth anatomy with emphasis on the interproximal areas has been advocated.[12]

It is also be possible to modify a thermoplastic template to permit the more accurate placement of resin composite to treat cases of anterior TW. One such protocol is that described by Mehta et al.,[14] termed the *resin injection moulding technique*, which may prove particularly helpful for the management of worn lower anterior teeth. This technique is summarised in Table 11.2.

The principles for the restoration of the worn anterior *mandibular dentition* are no different to those for the management of the worn antagonistic teeth, but, pragmatically, worn lower anterior teeth can give the treating clinician a few additional challenges, including the following:[14]

- Often, as a consequence of pathological TW, patients may present with rather diminutive lower front teeth with little remaining hard tissue.
- The lack of a sufficient quantity and quality of tooth enamel renders adhesive bonding somewhat unpredictable. Under such circumstances, there may be a need to undertake surgical crown-lengthening procedures and to consider the prescription of conventionally (mechanically) retained indirect restorations, such as crowns or overlays. Alternatively, the entire lingual surface could be used for bonding, resulting in wider and thicker lower anteriors ('oversized'), but with better retention and fracture strength.
- The freehand application of direct resin composite to restore worn lower teeth may also prove to be technically challenging, especially in cases of severe tooth surface loss.

Table 11.2 A summary of the resin injection moulding technique that can be used to restore worn lower anterior teeth.[14]

- Having verified the diagnostic wax-up, form an accurate stone duplicate onto which the PVC template will be fabricated. The thermoplastic stent most suitable for this purpose is of 0.5 mm thickness. Templates may be developed by either *vacuum forming* or *pressure forming*. The former is advocated, as the use of pressure to form the template can result in a relatively inflexible matrix, which may be difficult to prepare, place, and remove, and may be vulnerable to breakage of the stone cast.
- Once the stent has been adapted to the cast, trim the template using a pair of scissors. The template should extent past the second premolar teeth. Trim away excess material around the template margins. Gingivally, it is essential that there is at least 3–4 mm of material apical to the gingival margin to provide resilience. The template should be cut to follow a neat straight line, as opposed to a scalloped finish.
- With the template positioned on the cast, using a heated scalpel blade prepare slits in the template in the inter-proximal areas extending at least 3 mm apical to the contact area. It is imperative to use an adequately heated blade to ensure that neat incisions are produced without dragging the warmed template material when cutting. Verify the cuts made and remove any carbonised residue and debris with a pair of college tweezers.
- Place the sectioned matrix onto the *pre-operative cast*. Using a rugby ball-shaped diamond bur, make access vents into the template for each tooth that requires restoration. The vents should be placed approximately 3 mm coronal to the occlusal plane, on the facial aspect of the matrix. The access vent should be wide enough to permit the passive insertion of the tip of your chosen resin composite material.
- Prior to stent placement, floss the inter-proximal contacts and make a note of inter-proximal areas that may offer resistance to flossing. Try-in the modified template and check it for retention and stability. A poorly fitting template should be abandoned.
- Using a pair of scissors, cut 1.5 cm sections of a wide, straight steel matrix band. Ideally, a thin matrix should be used and four sections produced. With the template in situ, for each tooth to be treated attempt to place the sectioned matrices in each of the mesial and distal surfaces. Where this may prove challenging, review the stent to make sure that the slits have been correctly cut. If they are, minor inter-proximal reduction may need to be undertaken (with the patient's consent) using diamond polishing strips.
- Once you are satisfied that the matrices can be readily inserted and are retentive, remove the template. The choice can be taken to bevel the facial enamel and prepare a lingual butt margin. Any existing restorations should be assessed and replaced if deemed to be undesirable.
- For patients with moderate to advanced wear, if dentine needs to be replaced this can be accomplished by the formation of a *dentine cone*. Prior to tooth conditioning, prepare the teeth to improve the potential for micro-mechanical retention using either a slurry of oil-free pumice on a rubber cup or an air abrasion device. Protect the adjacent surfaces using an appropriate form of isolation. The choice may be taken to apply a split dam technique for effective tooth isolation. Apply the chosen adhesive protocol. Floss the inter-proximal contacts and cure as per the manufacturer's instructions.
- Using the chosen shade of dentine material, apply resin composite to form the dentine cones. The use of a fine-bladed inter-proximal carver is helpful for this task. The material should be finished to the inner surface of the labial bevel, allowing adequate space for an enamel layer. Light cure the layers of composite.
- Floss each of the inter-proximal areas. Remove any excess adhesive material with a sharp probe. Re-position the template and make sure that the matrix strips prepared earlier can be repositioned in the desired manner.

Table 11.2 (Continued)

- Select a tooth to restore. Re-condition this tooth for adhesive bonding, using isolation to protect the neighbouring teeth.
- Teeth should ideally be resorted on an individual basis (one at a time), but with experience of this technique multiple teeth can be restored.
- Place the matrices into the mesial and distal inter-proximal areas. The matrices should pass 3 mm apical to the contact area.
- For a right-handed operator, place the thumb of the left hand between the matrices; this will avoid excess material from flowing lingually, help to stabilise the template, and permit an improved adaptation of the matrices. Ideally, using pre-warmed resin, insert the resin compule into the access vent and carefully backflow resin composite into the matrix. Flowable resins are not advocated for this technique.
- Using a flat plastic instrument, apply gentle pressure to the template (in a labio-lingual direction) to improve adaptation. Remove excess material around the access vent, otherwise you risk locking the template in situ. Light-cure according to the manufacturer's instructions.
- Carefully remove the matrices and prize away the template. Inspect the resin augmentation. At this stage, any voids may be repaired by further resin additions. Resist adding bulk increments, otherwise the template will not re-seat
- Using a fine needle-shaped diamond bur, remove any flash excess. Caution must be applied to avoid removing excess material. Using an inter-proximal polishing strip in an S-shaped motion, to avoid the flattening and subsequent loss of patent of the inter-dental contacts, carefully remove excess material inter-proximally and round off any sharp corners at the line angles of the restored tooth.
- Repeat this procedure for the next tooth and continue until the injection moulding technique is completed. Using a set of composite finishing tungsten carbide burs, complete any gross finishing. A pointed cone shaped bur can be very helpful for completing the lingual surface, as well as the establishment of the required embrasure spaces. A flame-shaped bur can help with the refinement of the labial profile. You may choose to use an inter-dental bur to refine areas around the contact point.
- Verify the occlusal form using articulating foil and paper. Resin addition or subtraction may be undertaken until the desired aesthetic and functional parameters are derived. Fine polishing may be delayed to a subsequent session. Check the embrasure spaces, connectors, contact areas, and emergence profile to make sure you are satisfied with the overall contour.

- The use of a silicone index may also prove difficult where teeth are severely retroclined or in a patient with a shallow lingual sulcus and a raised tongue position.
- Effective moisture control can sometimes prove difficult for lower anterior teeth.

Figure 11.1 shows a case where the upper anterior localised worn dentition has been restored with direct composite.

11.3.2 Indirect Resin Composite Restorations

A number of differing treatment protocols have been described in the literature for the use of indirect resin restorations to treat TW, with variations relating to the extent of the restoration and the level of tooth preparation indicated (if any).

Satterthwaite[15] described the use of a direct/indirect technique involving the placement of *indirectly fabricated splinted palatal composite veneers* (with the palatal contour being fabricated in the dental laboratory) for the management of a case of anterior maxillary wear, with the labial aspect being undertaken free-hand using direct resin composite, where the longer-term plan was to prescribe subsequent crown restorations.

Mehta et al.[16] also documented the use of *indirectly fabricated resin overlays* for the management of anterior TW. Tooth preparation was confined to the removal of any sharp external line angles (for the purpose of reducing stress concentration post-cementation) and the inclusion of a knife edge/light chamfer margin to enable the dental technician to determine the finishing line. The use of 20 µm alumina blasting of the preparations was also undertaken, as advocated by Patel.[17] Post-cementation, the marginal appearance of indirect resin overlays can be enhanced by the addition of direct resin composite; this may be predictably bonded to the indirect restoration and residual dental hard tissues.

Acevedo et al.[18] described a treatment approach that involves the initial restoration of the worn anterior dentition using direct composite, followed by substitution with indirect resin veneers. A precision tooth preparation approach was taken (as recommended by Magne[19]) using a PVS index as a guide; depth reduction grooves were prepared and marked on the labial surface using a pencil. Veneers were cemented using a traditional approach, ensuring the preparation of the fit surface using sandblasting and silanisation.

A recent clinical trial comparing indirect and direct composite resin restorations for the treatment of severe TW on first molars demonstrated more fractures of indirect composite restorations compared to direct restorations. However indirect restorations showed less wear compared to direct restorations.[20] For anterior teeth that were restored with a combined lingual and buccal veneer technique, interfacial problems between these two parts of the restorations could be prevented when the restoration was directly placed in one session. It has been reported that repair techniques, including sandblasting and silane application, result in more adhesive problems then when a layering technique is used in one session.[10]

As material technology is improving, it is likely that superior results may become attainable using indirect resin composite. Indeed, a case report has been made available documenting the management of severe TW by minimal intervention using *CAD/CAM-generated high-density polymer restorations* for the pre-treatment of complex cases.[21]

11.3.3 Cast Metallic Restorations

The use of cast metal restorations to treat anterior TW is by no means a recent concept. Indeed, in 1975, Dahl et al.[22] described the use of a *removable anterior bite platform* fabricated from cobalt chromium retained by clasps in the canine and premolar regions to create inter-occlusal space in a patient with TW localised to the anterior maxillary segment. The appliance was designed to cover the cingulum rears of the affected teeth and increase the OVD in the region of 2–3 mm. The placement of this appliance culminated in posterior teeth disclusion, and occlusal contacts were only present between the mandibular anterior teeth and the bite platform. The appliance was prescribed for continual wear for several months until the posterior teeth re-established inter-occlusal contact.

Removal of the appliance resulted in an inter-occlusal space between the anterior maxillary and mandibular dentitions, which was subsequently utilised to restore the worn surfaces without the need for further tooth reduction.

However, given that compliance with removable appliances can be unpredictable, coupled with the display of unaesthetic clasps, Ibbetson and Setchel[23] described an alternative approach involving the prescription of a fixed-metal prosthesis to fulfil an analogous role, with the longer-term objective of replacing the castings with conventional indirect cast restorations. However, the following factors should be considered:

- The removal of the metallic backings may risk further compromising an already brittle dentition.
- The negative biological effects associated the preparation of such teeth to receive conventional restorations.
- The advent of chemically active resin luting cements that render the possibility of the formation of an effective and predictable bond between cast adhesive restorations and the dental hard tissues (thereby reducing the need for aggressive tooth preparations).
- Some patients may in fact consent to the provision of metallic restorations (due to the established merits as discussed in Chapter 10) for the restorations of non-aesthetic surfaces of anterior teeth.

The use of metal palatal veneers can provide an appropriate long-term restorative treatment option amongst some cases of anterior TW.

Type III gold alloy and alloys based on nickel-chromium (Ni-Cr) are the most commonly used alloys for the fabrication of fixed metallic adhesive restorations. Their relative merits are discussed in Chapter 10.

For anterior teeth, the preparation to receive a *metal palatal veneer* (also termed *palatal shims*) should include the removal of any undercuts and cover all remaining peripheral margins, extending up to the incisal edge, to optimise adhesive retention, aid placement, and improve resistance to shearing loads.[24] Pending material selection, an inter-occlusal clearance of between 0.5 and 1.5 mm is required. This may be attained through an ultra-conservative approach, whereby restorations are placed in supra-occlusion or by undertaking tooth preparation. In the former scenario, given the higher fracture resistance offered by cast metallic restorations (in contrast to resin composite or dental ceramics), the placement of supra-occlusal restorations can be undertaken with a higher level of confidence, especially amongst patients where high occlusal loading may be anticipated. Margins may be finished with either a knife edge or chamfer finish. The preparation of cingulum rests may also be useful, but preparation of the incisal edge should be avoided. Accurate impressions using a suitable gingival retraction protocol, appropriate (rigid and accurate) impressions trays, and a good-quality impression material are essential. Any required occlusal records should be taken to permit the use of an appropriate form of dental articulator (likely, a semi-adjustable device). Restorations should be waxed up and cast in accordance with the prescription, but where possible deep cingular areas should be avoided.

Type III gold restorations (Figure 11.2) require either heat treatment of the *fit surfa*ce, which may be carried out 400 °C for 4 minutes in an air furnace to form an active oxide layer, or tin plating of the fit surface to increase the surface energy to enhance bonding with resin cements. The combination of sandblasting and tin-plating has been described by Wada[25] to maximise resin retention to gold alloys. Tin-plating is thought to produce a roughened surface which will not only enable micro-mechanical retention but also chemical adhesion through the formation of hydrogen bonds with tin oxide. The internal surfaces of all metallic restoration should be sandblasted with 50 μm alumina (in the case of Type III gold alloy restorations, oxidation must be completed prior to sandblasting).

On receipt, metal veneers may be tried in using a calcium hydroxide paste, such as Dycal (Dentsply Ltd, Surrey, UK).[26] The inclusion of a metal tag or location lug is also helpful when trying-in/ cementing metal palatal veneer restorations. The latter may be readily removed with diamond burs and finished with a set of abrasive discs post-cementation.

Prior to carrying out cementation, effective isolation should be applied, ideally using a rubber dam. The surface to which the restoration is being bonded should be cleaned using either air abrasion or a slurry of oil-free pumice, and the veneers re-sandblasted (if required). The veneers should be cemented on an individual basis, using interproximal matrices to protect adjacent surfaces when undertaking the process of priming for adhesive bonding. The importance of using an appropriate alloy primer to ensure effective resin bonding is essential. The *dulling effect* of the metallic restoration, also commonly referred to in the literature as 'grey-out' or 'shine through', may be problematic. To some extent however, this may be partially masked by the use of opaque resins or by covering the labial surface with a tooth-coloured veneer. Where there may be a cosmetic concern with the display of metal from an adhesive onlay, sandblasting intra-orally post-cementation may help to reduce the visible gleam associated with this form of restoration.

Eliyas and Martin[26] described the use of gold palatal veneers to restore canine guidance (where the maxillary canine teeth are treated using metal veneers and the remaining maxillary anterior teeth are restored with direct resin composite) in two cases where rehabilitation utilising the Dahl concept was undertaken, where restoration of the incisal edge of the canine teeth may also be required. Under such circumstances, prior to veneer cementation, a bevel may be prepared on the incisal edge with a long shallow chamfer. Dry-retraction cord may also be used. Following the cementation of the veneer, the fit surface (to which resin composite will be applied to restore the incisal edge and mask the veneer) should be sandblasted and an opacious shade of resin composite and/or resin lute (such as Panavia 2.0F, Kuraray, Japan) applied to block out the dull metallic surface using a suitable alloy primer and resin composite applied accordingly.

This approach may be equally applied to restore worn posterior teeth.

11.3.4 Adhesive Ceramic Restorations

Dental ceramics may be broadly classified in accordance to their microstructure form, ranging from veneering ceramics to polycrystalline ceramics. The latter spectrum encompasses

- *glass ceramics/ veneering ceramics* (feldspathic porcelain and leucite)
- *glass ceramics with fillers* (lithium disilicate and alumina)
- *crystalline ceramics infiltrated with glass* (alumina-magnesia and alumina-zirconia)
- *polycrystalline ceramics* (polycrystalline alumina).[27]

Whilst veneering ceramics offer superior aesthetic value and the potential to be etched and micromechanically bonded to enamel and dentine, they have relatively low flexural strength, fracture toughness, and fracture strength, and require the support of either a metallic or high-strength ceramic core to help impart the necessary qualities to the definitive restorations (especially when applied to areas of higher occlusal loading).

Vailati et al.[28] described the use of *ceramic facial veneers* to provide treatment of labial surfaces as part of a technique termed the *sandwich approach*, whereby in cases with anterior maxillary wear the palatal surfaces are initially restored using a composite (direct or indirect) veneer. Preparation of the teeth to receive the ceramic veneers as per the authors' technique can be limited to the preparation of a light chamfer margin following the curvature of the gingiva, the rounding-off of all the line angles, immediate dentine sealing of any exposed dentine, and a butt joint preparation provided with the palatal veneer. On cementation, the *feldspathic veneers* must be etched with hydrofluoric acid, placed in alcohol, cleaned in an ultrasonic bath, treated with three coats of silane, and dried in an oven for about 1 minute at 100 °C, followed by the application of a coat of adhesive resin. Teeth should be air-abraded and the veneers bonded using a pre-warmed resin composite under rubber dam isolation. Patients with parafunctional tendencies should be provided with a post-operative nightguard.

The application of less invasive, *dentine-bonded crowns* may also have a promising role in the management of worn lower anterior teeth. Dentine-bonded crowns may be best described as an all-ceramic crown bonded to dentine (and any available enamel) using a resin-based luting material with the bond being mediated by the use of an adhesive bonding system and a micromechanically retentive ceramic surface. Effectively, the latter take the form of a complete porcelain veneer, whereby strength is derived by bonding to the underlying tissue.

Burke[29] published a case report describing the successful use of dentine-bonded crowns fabricated from feldspathic porcelain (treated by hydrofluoric acid) to treat a case of severe TW in a bulimic patient. Minimal tooth reduction was undertaken involving an occlusal clearance of 1.0 mm and preparations were finished with a knife-edged margin at gingival level.

Dentine-bonded crowns offer the merits of superior aesthetics (as they do not have a metal substructure or opaque porcelain sublayer), and the ability to bond to teeth has a considerable advantage in not only providing a patent marginal seal but where there has been copious loss of hard tooth tissue, particularly where the residual tooth structure has an over-tapered presentation. The latter forms of crown have also been reported to provide a satisfactory level of fracture resistance. However, the risks of fracture amongst patients who display parafunctional tooth-grinding habits must remain a concern. Their application is also costly and time-consuming, and such restorations are unsuitable where preparations extend subgingivally. It has been suggested that the presence of a gingival enamel ring is key to minimising their relative strength(s).

The use of *all-ceramic crowns* with a high-strength zirconia core has also been described amongst patients with TW.[30] As part of the author's treatment protocol, teeth were prepared to receive a circumferential chamfer finish placed at or slightly coronal to the gingival margin. Whilst axial reduction was carried out (to achieve a taper of 5–10°) together with the separation of the inter-proximal contacts, no occlusal reduction was provided. Cores were fabricated using CAD-CAM milling to ensure a thickness greater than 1 mm and subsequently layered using LAVA™ ceramic. Crowns were designed to minimise the effects of tensile and non-axial loading as well as to provide shallow and evenly shared anterior guidance (on mandibular protrusion) and thicker incisal edges, which was facilitated by the use of a semi-adjustable articulator. As part of the fitting process, the internal surfaces were roughened by sandblasting and cemented using a composite resin cement. Given that zirconia is not etchable, bonding with bisphenol A-glycidyl methacrylate (BisGMA) resins is likely to be less reliable. The use of a cement containing 10-methylacryl oxy decyl dihydrogen phosphate as the functional monomer may offer improved adhesion.[30]

11.3.5 Conventionally Retained Restorations

Conventionally retained indirect restorations are generally not advocated as the primary option for the management of the worn anterior dentition. However, they are sometimes prescribed (as discussed in Chapter 10) in cases where direct, adhesively retained materials may have been initially placed when carrying out rehabilitation using a reorganised approach to provide a short- to medium-term solution or where the patient may have consented to this type of care. The clinical techniques that can be applied to ensure predictability with conventional restorations when undertaking reorganised rehabilitation are discussed at length in Chapter 13.

Whilst details for the traditional prosthodontic protocols for the prescription of conventional crowns, onlays, and bridges can be found in any reputable textbook on fixed and removable prosthodontics, emphasis must be placed on the need for a *precision approach*, often involving the need for a diagnostic wax-up to prepare an appropriate silicone/acrylic indices to help guide tooth preparation, with the aim of conserving as much tissue as possible whilst concomitantly ensuring the requirement of the restorative material to yield optimal aesthetics and function.

In general, precious and non-precious metal alloys require a thickness of 0.7–1.5 mm, whilst metal-ceramic surfaces require 1.5 mm reduction on the labial surface(s) and 2.0–2.5 mm incisal reduction to ensure the required aesthetic, functional, and mechanical outcome.[27]

For cases of TW, additional considerations[31] when prescribing metal-ceramic crowns may include the following:

- Occlusal contacts in the ICP should (where possible) be prepared in metal, which is less abrasive towards an antagonistic natural dentition than porcelain.
- The porcelain–metal junction should be placed away from the occlusal contacts to avoid unwanted bending and sheer stresses that can otherwise result in ceramic fracture.
- The use of a metal collar to increase the rigidity if the metal substructure. A 0.7 mm chamfer margin will also reduce loss of cervical tissue, as opposed to a 1.2–1.5 mm shoulder margin.

The clinical protocols for the use of crown restoration are discussed further in Chapter 13.

11.4 Summary and Conclusions

In order to attain a successful outcome when embarking on the restorative rehabilitation of localised anterior TW, it is critical for the clinician to have a good understanding of the range of techniques that can be used to best manage the presenting problem.

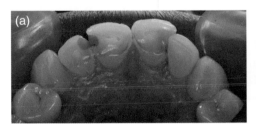
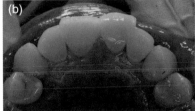

Figure 11.1 (a) Patient with localised anterior TW on the palatal surfaces of the upper canines, lateral and central incisors. (b) Patient shown in (a) with the anterior worn teeth restored with direct composite.

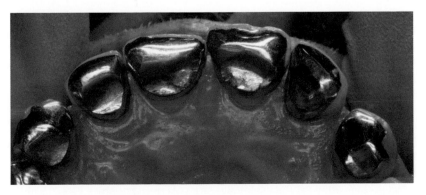

Figure 11.2 Patient with Type III gold alloy palatal veneers for localised anterior TW. This image shows the restorations at a 15-year recall appointment.

References

1 Mehta, S.B., Banerji, S., Millar, B.J., and Saures-Feito, J.M. (2012). Current concepts in tooth wear management. Part 2. Active restorative care 1: The management of localised tooth wear. *Br. Dent. J.* 212 (2): 73–82.

2 Chu, F., Botelho, M., Newsome, P. et al. (2002). Restorative management of the worn dentition 2. Localised anterior tooth wear. *Dent. Update* 29: 214–222.

3 Hemmings, K., Darbar, U., and Vaughan, S. (2000). Tooth wear treated with direct composite at an increased vertical dimension; results at 30 months. *J. Prosthet. Dent.* 83: 287–293.

4 Poyser, N., Porter, R., Briggs, P., and Kelleher, M. (2007). Demolition experts: management of the parafunctional patient 2. Restorative management strategies. *Dent. Update* 34: 262–268.

5 de Kok, P., Kleverland, C.J., Kuijs, R.H. et al. (2018 Feb). Influence of dentin and enamel on the fracture resistance of restorations at several thicknesses. *Am. J. Dent.* 31 (1): 34–38.

6 Burke, F. (2014). Information for patients undergoing treatment for toothwear with resin composite restorations placed at an increased occlusal vertical dimension. *Dent. Update* 41: 28–38.

7 Mehta, S.B., Banerji, S., Millar, B.J., and Saures-Fieto, J.M. (2012). Current concepts in tooth wear management. Part 4. An overview of the restorative techniques and materials commonly applied for the management of tooth wear. *Br. Dent. J.* 212 (4): 169–177.

8 Opdam, N., Skupien, J.A., Kreulen, C.M. et al. (2016). Case report: a predictable technique to establish occlusal contact in extensive direct composite resin restorations: the DSO technique. *Oper. Dent.* 41 (S7): S96–S108.

9 Hamburger, J., Opdam, N., Bronkhorst, E. et al. (2011). Clinical performance of direct composite restorations for treatment of severe tooth wear. *J. Adhes. Dent.* 13: 585–593.

10 Loomans, B.A.C., Kreulen, C.M., Huijs-Visser, H.E.C.E. et al. (2018). Clinical performance of full rehabilitations with direct composite in severe tooth wear patients: 3.5 years results. *J. Dent.* 70: 97–103.

11 Nixon, P., Gahan, M., and Chan, F. (2008). Techniques for restoring worn anterior teeth with direct composite resin. *Dent. Update* 35: 551–558.

12 Daoudi, M. and Radford, J. (2001). Use of a matrix to form directly applied resin composite to restore worn anterior teeth. *Dent. Update* 28: 512–514.

13 Mizrahi, B. (2004). A technique for simple and aesthetic treatment of anterior tooth wear. *Dent. Update* 31: 109–114.

14 Mehta, S.B., Francis, S., and Banerji, S. (2016). A guided, conservative approach for the management of localised mandibular anterior tooth wear. *Dent. Update* 43: 106–112.

15 Satterthwaite, J. (2012). Tooth surface loss: tools and tips for management. *Dent. Update* 39: 86–96.

16 Mehta, S.B., Banerji, S., Millar, B.J., and Saures-Fieto, J.M. (2012). Current concepts in tooth wear management. Part 3. Active restorative care 2: The management of generalised tooth wear. *Br. Dent. J.* 212 (3): 121–127.

17 Patel, M. (2016). Treating tooth surafe loss: restoration of the worn anterior dentition. *Prim. Dent. J.* 5 (3): 43–57.

18 Acevedo, R., Suarez-Feito, J., Tuero, C. et al. (2013). The use of indirect composite veneers to rehabilitate patients with dental erosion. *Eur. J. Esthet. Dent.* 8: 414–431.

19 Magne, P. and Belser, U. (2004). Novel porcelain laminate preparation driven by a diagnostic mock up. *J. Esthet. Rest. Dent.* 16: 7–16.

20 Loomans, B.A.C., Bougatsias, L., Sterenborg, B.A.M.M. et al. Survival of Direct and Indirect Composites Restorations in Toothwear Patients. IADR 2018, Abstract #0338.

21 Edelhoff, D., Beuer, F., Schweiger, J. et al. (2012). CAD/CAM-generated high-density polymer restorations for the pre-treatment of complex cases: a case report. *Quintessence Int.* 43: 457–467.

22 Dahl, B. and Krungstad, O. (1985). Long term observations of an increased occlusal face height obtained by a combined orthodontic/prosthetic approach. *J. Oral Rehabil.* 12: 173–170.

23 Ibbetson, R. and Setchell, D. (1989). Treatment of the worn dentition 2. *Dent. Update* 16: 300–307.

24 King, P.A. (1999). The use of adhesive restorations in the management of localised anterior tooth wear. *Prim. Dent. Care* 6 (2): 65–68.

25 Wada, T. (1986). Development of a new adhesive material and its properties. Proceedings of the International Symposium on Adhesive Prosthodontics, 9–19.

26 Eliyas, S. and Martin, N. (2013). The management of anterior tooth wear using gold palatal veneers in canine guidance. *Br. Dent. J.* 214: 291–297.

27 Ali, Z., Eliyas, S., and Vere, J. (2015). Choosing the right dental material and making sense of the options: evidence and clinical recommendations. *Eur. J. Prosthodont. Restor. Dent*: 151–162.

28 Vailati, F., Gruetter, L., and Belser, U. (2013). Adhesively restored anterior maxillary dentitons affected by severe erosion: up to 6-year results of a prospective clinical study. *Eur. J. Esthet. Dent.* 8: 506–528.

29 Burke, F. (1998). Treatment of loss of tooth substance using dentine bonded crowns: report of a case. *Dent. Update* 25: 235–240.

30 Milosevic, A. (2014). The survival of zirconia based crowns (Lava) in the management of severe anterior tooth wear up to 7-year follow-up. *Oral Biol. Dent.* 2: 1–7.

31 Poyser, N., Porter, R., Briggs, P., and Kelleher, M. (2007). Demolition experts: management of the parafunctional patient: 2. Restorative management strategies. *Dent. Update* 34: 262–268.

12

The Principles and Clinical Management of Localised Posterior Tooth Wear

12.1   Introduction

The principles for the management of localised posterior tooth wear (TW) in essence follow the same basic tenets as for localised anterior wear. Accordingly, having established the need for restorative intervention, there is a need to determine how inter-occlusal space will be provided to accommodate the chosen restorative material. Treatment options may include:

- the placement of the restoration in the existing inter-cuspal position (*conformative approach*) in cases where space may be present due to the rate of wear exceeding that of any dento-alveolar compensation or in the case of a missing anatagonistic tooth
- the *distalisation of the mandible*,[1] where any possible space between the inter-cuspal position and the first point of tooth contact in centric relation (CR) may permit the feasible placement of the restoration with the condyles further seated in the fossa
- the placement of the restoration in *supra-occlusion*, where there is a need to carefully assess the *eruptive potential* and condylar repositioning present as well assess the effects of placing a restoration in supra-occlusion on the surrounding hard and soft tissues
- undertaking of *substractive tooth preparation*.

For cases of early posterior TW, a *preventative approach* may be taken and may be all that is required. This may range from giving appropriate advice to the placement of suitable *sealant restorations* and/or the prescription of a *riser restoration* (assuming that TW is present at the surfaces involved in mandibular guidance) to reduce the risk of further wear at the affected tooth/teeth.

Restoration of the *worn posterior occlusal anatomy* may be undertaken using either a direct or indirect approach; restorations may be placed to conform to the existing occlusion (which may involve further subtractive tooth preparation) or be placed in a supra-occlusal position (with/or without a significant change being encountered with the patient's existing/physiological occlusal scheme).

Practical Procedures in the Management of Tooth Wear, First Edition. Subir Banerji, Shamir Mehta, Niek Opdam and Bas Loomans.
© 2020 John Wiley & Sons Ltd. Published 2020 by John Wiley & Sons Ltd.
Companion website: www.wiley.com/go/banerji/toothwear

The aim of this chapter is to appraise the techniques that may be used to undertake the restorative rehabilitation of the localised worn posterior dentition, commencing with the prescription of a preventative/riser restoration.

12.2   The Canine–Riser Restoration

The anatomy and location of the canine teeth, which commonly have a lengthy, bulbous root, renders them suitable for the process of providing posterior disclusion (Figure 12.1).[2] Wearing away of the occluding surfaces of the canine teeth can culminate in the failure of these teeth to provide effective *canine guidance*. Accordingly, there may be an indication to restore these surfaces:

- when attempting to prevent further TW (at relatively unaffected surfaces), where such surfaces may have in the past received 'canine protection' from an effective canine-guided occlusal scheme
- for the protection of restored surfaces (assuming the presence of some element of canine TW) from the effects of any destructive lateral loading during dynamic mandibular movements.

However, it should be noted that not everyone has canine guidance. Moreover, the protective value of canine guidance has never been proven in prospective studies and it mostly based on theories from 'traditional' prosthodiontic treatment concepts. Therefore, the indication for (re-)creating canine guidance has to be related to specific patient characteristics, such as a history of broken cusps in the posterior region, presence of active grinding, etc.

This form of restoration is sometimes also referred to as a *canine riser* or *Stuart lift* and has been postulated to work by altering the cuspal incline of the canine teeth to provide a canine-guided occlusion.[3] The clinical technique for the fabrication of such restoration(s) is summarised in Table 12.1.[4]

12.3   Techniques for the Restoration of Localised Posterior Wear Using Adhesively Retained Restorations

Restoration of the worn posterior tooth may involve the *bonding* of restorative material to the affected surfaces to provide the necessary form and function, or the placement of a more expansive restoration (often needing further tooth preparation). In the former scenario, *adhesive onlay restorations* (inclusive of occlusal veneers) can prove to be a very good treatment option (assuming the presenting circumstances favour effective adhesive dentistry). Each of the options will be appraised below.

12.3.1   Direct Composite Onlays

The direct application of resin composite overlays to attain the desired functional and morphological outcome demands operator skill (Figure 12.2). The prescription of direct resin onlays may prove highly valuable not only for the short-term

Table 12.1 Summary of the clinical stages involved with the fabrication of a canine-rise restoration.

- A complete occlusal assessment should be carried out.
- A long cone periapical radiograph be prescribed of the canine tooth/teeth to provide further insight into the morphology and size of the root, the level of alveolar support, the presence of any apical pathology (including root resorption), evidence of ankylosis, carious lesions, status of any existing restorations, and the morphology of the pulp chamber.
- Endodontically treated canine teeth, heavily restored or brittle canine teeth (as may be encountered in the geriatric patient) may be unsuitable for this form of restoration due to heightened risks of tooth fracture.
- A detailed periodontal analysis and aesthetic evaluation is also advisable.
- A mock-up riser by drying the tooth and placing resin composite (without any bonding) on the canine can be used as a means of attaining consent and allowing the patient to visualise the aesthetic outcome.
- The appropriate shade of resin composite is chosen. The centric stop on the canine tooth is identified and marked using articulating paper. This mark should ideally remain in situ during the course of the procedure.
- Following the implementation of an appropriate form of isolation, the enamel is cleaned using air abrasion or a slurry of oil-free pumice. Cleaning should be confined to the hard tissues superior to the centric stop, and should be extended over the incisal edge towards the facial surface.
- Isolation of the adjacent teeth is recommended to avoid inadvertent resin adhesion, and the tooth prepared for adhesive bonding.
- For a severely worn canine tooth a dentine shade of resin composite may be required along with the enamel shade, taking great care to only add material superior (incisal) to the marked centric stop. The inadvertent placement of composite resin on or inferior to (gingival) the centric stop will culminate in an increase the patient's occlusal vertical dimension.
- The dentine shade is added in a manner to restore the dentine tissue which has been lost and light-cured. The resin should be placed in increments no greater than 2.0 mm to permit adequate curing.
- The selected enamel shade is placed to restore the enamel layer. The enamel layer should be extended onto the facial surface to cover as much of the labial enamel as possible without compromising the aesthetic or oral hygiene requirements of the patient. After light-curing the enamel layer, a final translucent layer of resin composite may be applied.
- The efficacy of the restoration placed should be evaluated. Ideally it should provide canine guidance, which can be verified by asking the patient to demonstrate a lateral excursive movement, which should result in disclusion on both the working and non-working side. Articulating paper can be used to aid the verification process.
- Further increments of resin can be applied if required. The ramp provided should harmonise with the residual occlusion, otherwise displacement and/or mobility of the canine teeth will result.
- Finishing and polishing may be carried out as described above.
- The inter-proximal contacts should be flossed and any unwanted adhesive removed accordingly. Caution must be taken with the finishing and polishing protocol to make sure that the ability of the restoration to provide posterior disclusion is maintained and wear of the opposing teeth is minimised.

The technique described here relates to the placement of resin composite in a *direct manner* to restore a worn maxillary canine, but it can be equally applied to restore a worn mandibular canine tooth, or perhaps both, dependant on the level of wear observed and the aesthetic demands of the patient.

protection of worn posterior surfaces as *intermediate composite resin restorations*, to determine a patient's tolerance to a planned change in their occlusal scheme (with minimal intervention and optimal contingency planning), but to also provide protection to recently placed anterior restorations, which may otherwise be susceptible to failure from increased occlusal loading.

There are a number of restorative techniques that have been described for the placement of direct composite to restore the worn posterior occlusal anatomy, including:

- freehand application of material
- direct shaping by occlusion (DSO)
- use of a silicone index formed from a wax-up
- use of a vacuum-formed matrix template.

In general, however, when attempting to provide an indirect posterior resin onlay there needs to be at least 1.5 mm of inter-occlusal clearance in areas of loading. When using a direct composite resin restoration, the minimal thickness is less important.

For the *freehand placement of resin composite* (which may sometimes be indicated as an intermediate restoration), in an attempt to ascertain the tolerance of the patient to a potenital supra-occlusal restoration, the resin overlay can be finished to a 'flat' occlusal morphology. Once the patient has displayed acceptance, the resin onlay may be substituted with a more robust material or a new direct resin restoration with more anatomical form/features that can be done with minimal further tooth reduction (as the required occlusal clearance will have been provided by the process of relative axial movement). When prescribing direct restoration to establish tolerance in the manner described, it may be appropriate to keep the restoration clear of occlusal contact during dynamic mandibular movements by the addition of a riser restoration. If the guiding tooth has signs of wear, a riser may be retained in the longer term. However, if there are no signs of wear present, the riser should be removed following the establishment of occlusal contacts. This technique has been described for the successful management of symptomatic, cracked teeth with incomplete tooth fracture(s).[5] This technique can also be used to treat patients with localised (severe) wear on posterior teeth and functional problems (such as pain during eating). It is a minimally invasive approach to restoratively treat teeth that present clinical signs of discomfort.

An alternative is to use the *DSO technique*.[6] This technique facilitates the shaping of a restoration and helps to obtain the occlusion in the desired dimension. The essential part of this technique is that the final increment of composite resin covering the occlusal or palatal surface is left uncured when the patient is asked to occlude, after which the composite resin is cured.

For generalised TW, this restorative technique starts with the lower anterior teeth, which are restored freehand. When the lower anterior teeth are shaped and finished, sufficient space must be left between the restored lower incisors and the unrestored upper anterior teeth with stops in situ (see Chapter 11) in order to allow restoration of their palatal surfaces. After finishing and polishing the lower anterior teeth, a metal matrix band is inserted from the palatal side of a central upper incisor and secured with wooden wedges. Before placing the matrix, the estimated height of the metal should be adjusted with scissors. After placement, the matrix band can be adjusted again using a high-speed diamond bur. Finally, when the patient closes onto the stops there should be no interference between matrix and antagonists. Although intentionally no rubber dam is applied, appropriate moisture control is achieved using an Optragate (Ivoclar Vivadent) device and additional cotton rolls, a suction device, a proper matrix, wedge placement and a chairside dental nurse.

The first cervical layer of restorative composite is placed and cured up to a level 1 mm below the matrix. Subsequently, the final layer of the restorative composite is inserted to cover the entire surface inside the matrix being sufficient for the antagonistic teeth to make a clear impression in the uncured composite. This layer is left uncured, whilst the antagonistic tooth is either covered with a layer of Teflon foil or coated with a thin film of glycerine jelly. The patient is asked to close onto the stops, resulting in an impression of the lower anterior teeth in the uncured composite. After curing for at least 40 seconds with a powerful light-curing unit, the patient is asked to open and the composite is additionally post-cured from different directions. In many cases the vestibular surface is subsequently restored with a direct composite veneer, using an anterior composite in a multi-layer technique and finally the first tooth is finished and polished. All upper anterior teeth are reconstructed in a similar way, whilst the posterior stops are kept in situ during closing in order to ensure identical occlusal vertical dimension (OVD).

Once the reconstruction of the maxillary upper front teeth is complete, the posterior teeth are reconstructed using the same procedure. The sequence of restoration is as follows:

1) Upper first premolars are built up freehand in the estimated curve of Spee in line with the upper canines.
2) The lower first premolars are restored using DSO.
3) The lower posterior teeth are built up in the estimated right plane prior to restoring the upper antagonists, leaving sufficient space for building up those teeth.
4) The upper second premolars and molars are restored using DSO.

As with the reconstruction of the anterior teeth, the occlusal surfaces are finished and interferences in lateral excursions are removed using fine grit diamond burs, aiming at contact in occlusion and preserving canine guidance.

A *diagnostic wax-up* can also be used to form a silicone key and can be used as a guide to the height of the occlusal table. This can help to re-establish the tooth morphology and functional occlusion. Accordingly, a restorative protocol has been described by Ramseyer et al., referred to as the *stamp technique*, which warrants further exploration.[7] Silicone templates, *stamps*, are made of the wax-up using a smooth surface silicone material (in the authors' case, President Putty Soft, Coltene, Whaledent, Switzerland). The set index can then be sectioned into a *vestibulat part* and *oral part* for each tooth. Having carried out isolation using a rubber dam and prepared the teeth for adhesive bonding (inclusive of the replacement of any metallic or failed restorations with resin composite, the roughening of dentine with a diamond bur for 15 seconds, and the placement of sectional inter-proximal matrices), one of the sections can be loaded with the chosen resin composite material and placed at a 45° angle onto the lateral surface of the tooth; the unwaxed surfaces are used as a guide to ensure correct placement of the matrix. Following the adaptation of the material against the index and tooth, the stamp is carefully removed by applying a rolling motion towards the contralateral side of the tooth. Following the removal of excess material, light-curing is performed for 20 seconds and the process repeated using the second stamp. Gross finishing may be carried out prior to the departure of the patient, but the final finishing and polishing stages are better undertaken during a subsequent appointment.

The use of a *vacuum-formed matrix template* to restore the worn posterior dentition using direct composite resin restorations has been described by Schmidlin et al.[8] As an extrapolation of their protocol, all existing metal-based restorations should be replaced with resin composite materials, and any existing dental caries managed accordingly. A duplicate cast is then made of the wax-up, upon which a vacuum-formed matrix is prepared. To ensure stability of the matrix, the front teeth and the most distal tooth should not be waxed-up, and the template made to fit around their worn surfaces. Under the influence of local anaesthesia and rubber dam isolation, small metal matrices can be placed in the inter-proximal areas (to ensure that unwanted material does not become trapped) in these areas. Existing resin restorations should be air abraded and the enamel tissues etched for 120 seconds using 35% phosphoric acid. Following the preparation of the teeth for effective adhesive bonding, notably undertaken in an alternative manner, the matrix can be filled with a hybrid resin composite-based material and placed onto the tooth surfaces. With the matrix in situ, the material should be light-cured for 3–4 seconds. The template may then be carefully removed, along with any excess material. The restorations (as per the author's protocol) should be light-cured for 60 seconds and gross finishing undertaken. The untreated teeth may then be restored analogously, and the distal tooth built up using a freehand method.

With this technique, air entrapment, ensuring the effective adaptation of the material to the tooth surface, proper proximal contacts, and the complication of unset material (given that large increments may be placed) can be problematic factors.

12.3.2 Indirect Adhesive Onlay Restorations

Onlay restorations may be *conventionally retained* (by means of macro-mechanical retention form) or retained by a combination of chemical and micro-mechanical adhesion (*adhesive onlay*) (Figure 12.3). The merits if adhesive onlays are alluded to in Chapter 10.

Indirect adhesive onlays may be fabricated using *composite resin, metallic alloys* or *ceramic*.

For the placement of a *cobalt chromium onlay*, Yap[9] described a conservative preparation that requires an occlusal clearance of 1.0 mm on the functional cusp bevel and 0.7 mm on the non-functional cusps (given the extreme rigidity of chromium alloys), and the buccal, distal, and lingual margins placed 1.2 mm beneath the (prepared) occlusal surface. The margins should be finished with a shoulder design. It may be best to replace existing metal restorations (as well as manage existing carious lesions) using resin composite. The marginal finish line should extend 0.5 mm apical to any restorative material, ideally terminating on enamel tissue.

For a *Type III or IV cast gold alloy restoration*, there will be a need to be an inter-occlusal clearance of 1.0–1.5 mm on the non-functional and functional cusps respectively, with the buccal, palatal, and axial margins placed 1.2 mm (with a chamfer margin/bevelled/bevelled shoulders) circumferentially below the prepared occlusal surface.[9,10]

For *ceramic onlay restorations*, there the manufacturer's instructions should be followed to avoid premature failure, but up to 2.0 mm of inter-occlusal clearance is often advocated, concomitantly ensuring that all of the internal line angles are rounded and walls divergent occlusally with the absence of any grooves or sharp angles.[11]

However, the use of minimally invasive tooth preparations using monolithic lithium disilicate posterior occlusal veneers (without any veneering porcelain) has been described by Fradeani et al.[12] (for the restoration of posterior TW), ensuring an occlusal thickness of 0.8–1.0 mm, finished with a chamfer margin and with overall inter-occlusal clearance of 0.8 mm on the occlusal surface and 0.4–0.6 mm on the axial surfaces.

Space for onlay restorations may be provided by either undertaking tooth preparation involving the need to prescribe the above levels of inter-occlusal clearance or placement in a supra-occlusal location to that of the existing plane. In the latter scenario, marginal preparation should be undertaken as described above. Consideration also needs to be given to sandwich-type indirect restorations where the path of insertion can be altered to minimise tooth reduction.

For the use of *indirect resin composite materials* to treat posterior wear (to take advantage of the merits of resin composite as a restorative material, as discussed in Chapter 9), where the use of direct materials may prove technically more challenging (especially amongst cases of more advanced toot tissue loss), the use of indirect resin onlays fabricated using conventional laboratory techniques or 3D CAD/CAM (Lava Ultimate, 3M ESPE) has been described in the literature, with little tooth preparation is advocated.[13,14] However, to ensure longevity, the onlays should be of an appropriate minimal thickness (at least 1.5 mm). In both cases, a silicone key is made from the wax-up to guide the placement of the onlays. Metal matrices are inserted inter-proximally and an impression taken (with the matrices captured within the impression), yielding open contact points on the cast to aid fabrication of the restorations. Cementation is undertaken by the placement of the onlay into a clear silicone index (Elite Transparent, Zhermack) formed from the pre-operative wax-up, and the onlays are loaded with a chosen shade of pre-warmed resin composite and pressed against the worn surfaces. The use of a clear silicone material offers the advantage of allowing the operator to undertake light-curing/polymerisation with the index in place. Excess resin can then be removed before completing the cementation stage.

The fabrication of a provisional restoration for an adhesive onlay can prove challenging. Where a diagnostic wax-up is available, it may be indexed and a custom direct provisional restoration formed using a bis-acryl based temporary crown and bridge material. Restorations may be cemented using zinc polycarboxylate cement or a eugenol-free temporary cement (such as Temp-Bond NE, Kerr).

In the absence of a wax-up, a direct provisional restoration may be fabricated; accordingly, the adjacent teeth should be isolated using a circumferential matrix band. Acid etch (37% orthophosphoric acid, no more than two spots) can be placed on the buccal and palatal/lingual surfaces apical to the marginal finish line. Some clinicians also elect to apply a dentine bonding agent, which will also help to immediately form a dentine seal;[15] resin composite may then be applied and extended to the etched area.

To take appropriate working impressions, the use of a putty and wash impression system is perhaps better avoided, as the putty can displace the wash material away from the marginal area, culminating in the critical marginal area being recorded in the less accurate material. When fabricating the onlay restoration, the dental technician should also be instructed to keep any die spacer away from the margins when forming the die stone.

The fit surface(s) may also require special attention (pending the material selected), as discussed in relation to adhesive metal/adhesive ceramic veneers used to restore the worn anterior teeth, in order to ensure adequate adhesion with the resin-based cement.

Cementation of the adhesive onlay(s) should ideally take place under rubber dam isolation. It is prudent to also isolate the adjacent teeth when preparing teeth for resin bonding to avoid inadvertent adhesion with resin lute during the cementation space.

12.4   Restoration of Localised Posterior Wear Using Conventionally Retained Restorations

In general, the use of conventionally retained indirect (crown and onlay) restorations for the treatment of posterior TW may range from the management of a single tooth to multiple teeth. In either case, it is imperative to apply established restorative protocols in order to ensure the desired functional (occlusal) outcome. Additional clinical techniques/stages may also need to be undertaken where, for instance, the affected tooth/teeth may be the first point of contact in centric relation, or be involved with the provision of mandibular guidance. The generic treatment protocols in relation to the latter are discussed further below.

The details in relation to the undertaking of crown and onlay preparations (including the process of undertaking precision tooth reduction, the recording of impressions, the making of provisional restorations, and soft tissue management in the area of treatment provision) are generally well appraised in any reputable text on fixed and removable prosthodontics.

12.5   Management of the Occlusal Scheme When Using Indirect Restorations to Treat Localised Posterior TW (Other than in the Supra-Occlusal Location)

12.5.1   The Conformative Approach with Indirect Restorative Techniques

In the case of a single unit posterior crown/onlay, where the affected tooth is not involved in providing any forms of mandibular guidance during any lateral excursive or protrusive movements and does not carry the first point of contact in centric relation (CR), the retruded contact position (RCP), following the process of completing the tooth preparation, the use of hand-held casts to fabricate the restoration may be deemed sufficient; accordingly, an inter-cuspal (ICP) record may be taken (if required) as discussed in Chapter 5.[16]

When trying-in and fitting the definitive restoration, it is important to verify that the centric stops pre-and post-cementation are of the coincident variety, with patent holding contacts elucidated, using a section of appropriately supported Shimstock foil (analogous to the processes described for direct restoration).

When providing a limited number of *multiple posterior restorations* (three units or less, which may also include bridgework) where the teeth will not be involved in providing mandibular guidance (such as for a patient displaying a canine-guided occlusal scheme), it is sensible to attain a facebow record as well as an ICP record to enable the use of either an average value articulator or a semi-adjustable articulator, where average values may be applied to programme the device for parameters such as the *intercondylar width*, the *incisal guidance angle*, the *Condylar guidance angle*, the *Bennet angle* (*progressive side shift*) and the *immediate side shift* (*Bennet movement*), as described in Chapter 5.[16] This will hopefully provide the dental technician with further information on how to best develop the anatomical form of the restorations in relation to features such as *cusp height*, *cusp angles* and the placement of *cusp tips and grooves.*

When preparing multiple teeth, to maintain reference points it may be sensible to prepare alternative teeth at different visits and/or by obtaining an ICP record immediately following the preparation of some teeth by interposing a dimensionally stable registration medium (as an appropriate form of PVS bite registration material or a cold-cured acrylic) between the opposing occluding surfaces in the inter-cuspal position. This can then be used to mount the working cast against the opposing pre-mounted study cast.

However, if it is established that the given posterior tooth/teeth does/do indeed have a critical role in providing guidance and there is the desire to preserve or 'copy' this function into the definitive indirect restoration, then a set of accurate pre-operative study casts should be fabricated, a facebow record taken, and, if necessary, a record of the inter-cuspal position also obtained.

Using these records, the diagnostic/pre-definitive restoration casts can be mounted on a semi-adjustable articulator in the inter-cuspal position. A *customised incisal guidance table* (also sometimes referred to as an *anterior guidance table* or an *incisal bite table*) should then be fabricated.[17] The latter has been defined as a device 'used for transferring to an articulator the contacts of anterior teeth when determining their influence on border movements of the mandible' and can be used to 'copy' the occlusal prescription and features of the guiding surfaces, thereby preserving the desired dynamic occlusal scheme.[18] The technical stages involved with the fabrication of the latter device include the following:[17]

a) Mounting a set of pre-definitive restoration casts onto a semi-adjustable articulator.

b) Raising the incisal pin of the articulator by approximately 1.5–2 mm.

c) Lightly coating the tip of the incisal pin with petroleum jelly (to act as a separator)

d) An appropriate quantity of cold cured acrylic should be mixed according to the manufacturer's instructions and when at the 'doughy' stage the material should be transferred to the incisal guidance table. There are a variety of cold-cured acrylic materials that can be used for this purpose.

e) Whilst the acrylic material is still setting, the tip of the incisal pin should be transcribed through the material by moving the upper member of the articulator backwards and from side to side, thereby guiding the incisors through simulated excursive and protrusive movements. In this way, a record will have been made of the articulator during dynamic movements.

f) Once set, it is important to verify the that the incisal pin has formed a patent contact with the registration material (thereby ensuring that the ICP record has been maintained). This can be checked using a piece of suitably supported Shimstock articulating foil.

g) The table can be carefully trimmed to remove any excess, without compromising the record, concomitantly permitting optimal visualisation of the movements of the tip of the pin whilst making sure it remains in contact with the acrylic-based table.

h) The working cast can now be mounted against the antagonistic pre-existing cast (using an inter-cuspal record if necessary).

i) The customised incisal guidance table can now be used to fabricate the definitive restoration, applying the record of the pre-restorative envelope of mandibular movement to determine the desirable crown height, length, and anatomy of the guiding surfaces. In an analogous manner, it is important to ensure that the incisal pin remains in contact with the guidance table in the appropriate manner, which can be verified using Shimstock foil as well as GHM articulating paper.

12.5.2 The Management of a Posterior Tooth Carrying the First Point of Contact in CR, the RCP

When the mandible is closed in the retruded arc of closure the first point of tooth contact is referred to the RCP. A clinical decision will have to be made as to whether to replicate this contact in the indirect restoration. Consideration needs to given to the material choice in these circumstances to optimise the load-bearing capacity of the material if this contact is to be replicated. If it has been decided that this contact will be replicated in the restoration then prior to the reduction of the tooth the upper and lower dental casts for the patient are mounted onto a semi-adjustable articulator using a facebow and retruded (CR) arc of closure records. The pin of the articulator is loosened and the RCP is identified. Starting from this position an anterior guidance table is fabricated as described earlier. The teeth are brought forward into contact in the inter-cuspal and lateral movements are made to fabricate the guidance table. Once this has been achieved, the working cast can be mounted onto the articulator and the indirect cast restoration fabricated using the prescription as outlined by the customised guidance table.

12.6   Summary and Conclusions

In order to attain a successful outcome when embarking on the restorative rehabilitation of localised posterior TW, it is critical for the clinician to have a good understanding of the range of techniques and concepts that may be used to optimally manage the presenting pathology.

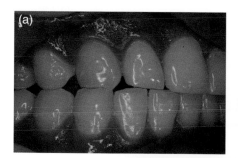
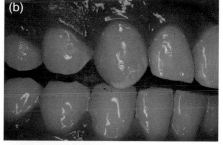
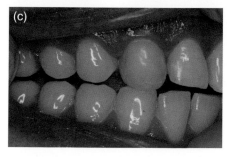

Figure 12.1 (a) The contact between the patient's upper and lower right teeth during lateral excursion to the patient's right-hand side. The working side contacts can be seen. (b) The right lateral excursion following a direct composite canine rise restoration placed on the upper right canine tooth for the patient shown in (a). Note the disclusion of the surrounding teeth as compared to the image in (a). (c) The wear of the direct composite canine rise restoration on the upper right canine for the patient shown in (a) and (b) at a 9-year recall appointment following placement of the restoration. Note the proximity of the surrounding teeth on the right lateral excursion following the wear of the direct composite.

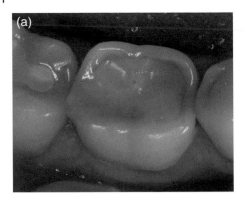
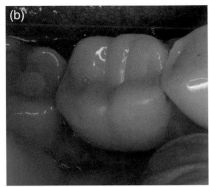

Figure 12.2 (a) Patient with a worn and sensitive lower right first molar tooth. (b) The lower right first molar tooth shown in (a) has been restored with direct composite and this view is at a recall appointment.

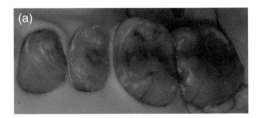
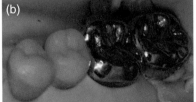

Figure 12.3 (a) Patient with TW. (b) Patient shown in (a) with the premolars restored with lithium disilicate and molars restored with gold alloy onlays immediately after cementation.

References

1 Yule, P. and Barclay, S. (2015). Worn down by toothwear? Aetiology, diagnosis and management revisited. *Dent. Update* 42: 525–532.
2 Eliyas, S. and Martin, N. (2013). The management of anterior tooth wear using gold palatal veneers in canine guidance. *Br. Dent. J.* 214: 291–297.
3 Murray, M., Brunton, P., Osborne-Smith, K., and Wilson, N. (2001). Canine risers: indcations and techniques for their use. *Eur. J. Prosthodont. Restor. Dent.* 9 (3–4): 137–140.
4 Banerji, S., Mehta, S.B., and Ho, C.K. (2017). *Practical Procedures in Aesthetic Dentistry*. Wiley Blackwell.
5 Banerji, S., Mehta, S.B., Kamran, T. et al. (2014). A multi-centred clinical audit to describe the efficacy of direct supra-coronal splinting – a minimally invasive approach to the management of cracked tooth syndrome. *J. Dent.* 42: 862–887.
6 Opdam, N., Skupien, J.A., Kreulen, C.M. et al. (2016). Case report: a predictable technique to establish occlusal contact in extensive direct composite resin restorations: the DSO-technique. *Oper. Dent.* 41 (S7): S96–S108.

7 Ramseyer, S., Helbling, C., and Lussi, A. (2015). Posterior vertical bite reconstructions of erosively worn dentitions and the "stamp technique" – a case series with a mean observation time of 40 months. *J. Adhes. Dent.* 17: 283–289.

8 Schmidlin, P., Filli, T., Imfeld, C. et al. (2009). Three tear evaluation of posterior vertical bite reconstruction using direct resin composite – a case series. *Oper. Dent.* 34: 102–108.

9 Yap, A. (1995). Cuspal coverage with resin bonded metal onlays. *Dent. Update* 22 (10): 403–406.

10 Chana, H., Kelleher, M., Briggs, P., and Hooper, R. (2000). Clinical evaluation of resin bonded gold alloy veneers. *J. Prosthet. Dent.* 83: 294–300.

11 Summitt, J., Robbins, J., Hilton, T. et al. (2006). *Fundamentals of Operative Dentistry, A Contemporary Approach*, 3e. Quintessence Books.

12 Fradeani, M., Barducci, G., Bacherini, L., and Brennan, M. (2012). Esthetic rehabilitation of a severely worn dentition with minimally invasive prosthetic procedures (MIPP). *Int. J. Periodontics Restorative Dent.* 32: 135–147.

13 Bartlett, D. and Sundaram, G. (2006). An up to 3 year randomised clinical study comparing indirect and direct resin composite used to restore worn posterior teeth. *Int. J. Prosthodont.* 19: 613–617.

14 Vailati, F. and Carciofo, S. (2016). CAD/CAM monolithic restorations and full mouth adhesive rehabilitation to restore a patient with a past history of bulimia: the modified three-step technique. *Int. J. Esthet. Dent.* 11: 36–56.

15 Hironaka, N., Ubaldini, A., Sato, F. et al. (2018). Influence of immediate dentine sealing and interim cementation on the adhesion of indirect restorations with dual polymerzing resin cement. *J. Prsothet. Dent.* 119 (4): 678, e1–678.e8.

16 Wassell, R., Naru, A., Steele, J., and Nohl, F. *Applied Occlusion. Quintessentials of Dental Practice – 29, Prosthodontics-5*, 2e. Quintessence Publishing.

17 Davies, S., Gray, R., and Whitehead, S. (2001). Good practice in advanced restorative dentistry. *Br. Dent. J.* 191: 421–434.

18 The Glossary of Prosthodontic Terms, Ninth Edition, GPT-9 (2017). The Academy of Prosthodontics Foundation. *J. Prosthet. Dent.* 117 (5S): e1–e105.

13

The Principles and Clinical Management of Generalised Tooth Wear

13.1   Introduction

The protocols for the technical execution of dental restorations for the treatment of severe tooth wear (TW) are analogous to those described in the previous two chapters, see flowchart (Figure 13.1). Accordingly, the focus of this section will be aimed at discussing the *principles for the management of generalised TW* (Figure 13.2).

For patients who may be affected by the process of generalised TW (as discussed in Chapter 6), there *may* also be a concomitant alteration in their *occlusal vertical dimension (OVD)*. The extent to which the latter may take place will depend largely on the level of impending dento-alveolar compensation. Consequently, it has become commonplace to consider the alteration in the OVD when planning restorative rehabilitation.

In relation to generalised TW it is clinically difficult to divide patients into groups as patient types as has been described by Turner and Missirilian:[1]

- *Category 1:* Excessive wear with loss of vertical dimension of occlusion
- *Category 2:* Excessive wear without loss of vertical dimension, but with space available
- *Category 3:* Excessive wear without loss of vertical dimension, but with limited space.

The above classification has indeed been used to help plan prosthodontic rehabilitation. An alternative pragmatic method has also been described for the management of patients where an increase in the OVD is required and one such protocol has been used as part of the *Radboud Tooth Wear Project* (Nijmegen, the Netherlands)[2] and will be considered in further detail as part of this chapter.

Regardless of the pattern of occlusal change associated with a dentition displaying generalised wear amongst cases where active intervention is being sought, a set of accurate diagnostic casts mounted in centric relation (CR) is strongly advocated.[3] Although a semi-adjustable articulator with an arbitrary face bow may be considered to be acceptable, if necessary, a kinematic transverse horizontal axis facebow transfer can help a tentative increase in the OVD without introducing errors in with horizontal jaw relationship. The true anatomical transverse horizontal axis may be different from that determined with the use of an arbitrary facebow.[4] In such cases an alteration in the OVD will result in a

Practical Procedures in the Management of Tooth Wear, First Edition. Subir Banerji, Shamir Mehta, Niek Opdam and Bas Loomans.
© 2020 John Wiley & Sons Ltd. Published 2020 by John Wiley & Sons Ltd.
Companion website: www.wiley.com/go/banerji/toothwear

loss of accuracy in the horizontal jaw relationship, possibly leading to erroneous restorations.[3] In the authors' opinion the use of such apparatus is also dependent upon the material of choice for the restorations proposed. If an adjustable material, for example composite, is used directly onto the patient's dentition and a period of occlusal adaptation can be observed to confirm the occlusal prescription with any necessary adjustments possible, then the use of a complex fully adjustable apparatus is not required. Once the occlusal prescription is confirmed in situ then individual or groups of teeth can have definitive restorations placed as required in a conformative rehabilitation process, as described later in this chapter.

In general, the desired increase in OVD will be primarily determined by (i) the amount and location of TW, (ii) the need to provide enough space for the restorations, and (iii) the need to and possibility of lengthening the anterior teeth.

Clinically, the freeway space can be estimated by undertaking a measurement of the existing OVD of the worn dentition and the face height with the mandible at rest with an adequate lip seal – the difference between the two measurements gives an indication of the existing freeway space and may possibly give an indication of the desired increase in the OVD, but in the authors' opinion the freeway space is not the most important factor as it will adapt after treatment. The determination of the freeway space is a subjective process due to the mobility of soft tissues overlying the extra-oral structures, as well as the limitations associated with the commonly available recording apparatus. Furthermore, the rest position of the mandible is also variable, being influenced by a number of factors such as speech, emotion, jaw relationships, alveolar bone resorption, body position, loss of natural tooth contacts, and the use of some prescription and recreational drugs.[5]

Together with these observations, the required increase in OVD is planned on the dental articulator (by raising the incisal pin on the articulator) based on the anticipated reconstruction of the anatomical form of the teeth, carefully considering the necessary inter-occlusal space posteriorly and anteriorly. According to the lip-generated smile design,[6] an intra-oral mock-up is designed using direct composite placement on teeth #13 to #23 without any enamel and/or dentine bonding procedures to check the new aesthetics with the patient. After approval of form and colour by the patient, the mock-up is recorded photographically for documentation and removed. If desired (e.g. for an indirect procedure or the production of a mould) a diagnostic wax-up can be fabricated accordingly (preferably on duplicate casts).[3] The intra-oral mock-up of the anterior teeth will then be the guideline for a diagnostic wax-up. The clinical processes for developing a functional-aesthetic dental wax-up, followed by the carrying out of an intra-oral mock-up to help attain informed consent, are discussed at length in Chapter 8.

Based on the authors' experience, the transfer of the planned increase in OVD (as determined by the mock-up and wax-up) to the patient's dentition should (ideally) be in the first instance done by technical processes that require minimal intervention and using materials that offer the scope and adjustment (by addition or subtraction, such as resin composite) to enable the evaluation of the patient's tolerance of the functional and aesthetic outcomes of the planned proposed changes. Once the latter have been ascertained (and the prescription accepted), then these restorations may be substituted by more robust dental materials (in the event of a need arising). Indeed, according to Loomans et al.,[7] restorative techniques should be as conservative as possible, including the treatment of the minimum number of teeth necessary in order to attain the desired clinical outcome. Where tooth preparation is required, it is suggested that this is of a minimally invasive nature to help facilitate restoration placement.

The above *phased* approach will not only permit an appropriate period of time to evaluate tolerance of the changes but may also help to avoid the propagation of potential errors which can sometimes arise where multiple units of more invasive restorations are prescribed (such as crowns) and where there may be marked changes to the patient's dentition from the status quo, especially where provisional restorations may not have been made best use of (as discussed further below).

The phasing of treatment in this manner may also help avoid the high initial financial cost associated with the prescription of multiple units of fixed indirect prosthodontic restorations, but the longer-term fees may prove to be higher, hence the need for appropriate patient communication and the attainment of informed consent at the outset (Figure 13.3).[3]

13.2 The Prosthodontic Approach to the Restorative Rehabilitation of Generalised Tooth Wear

The subclassification of cases of generalised TW by Turner and Missirilian[1] has been alluded to above. This classification may be helpful when planning restorative rehabilitation and is discussed below. It should be noted that there are not strict guidelines as the loss of OVD cannot be determined easily.

13.2.1 Category 1: Excessive tooth wear, together with a loss in the OVD

These cases are sometimes considered to be the least demanding of all three categories of generalised wear to manage, as the resultant inter-occlusal clearance created through the process of TW itself will provide most, if not all, the required inter-occlusal space for the restorative material, without the need for aggressive occlusal reduction (by a planned increase in the OVD).[8]

Whilst for many cases of generalised TW the fabrication of a full-coverage, hard acrylic stabilisation splint such as a Michigan splint (as described in Chapter 8) has traditionally been undertaken to evaluate a patient's tolerance/adaptability to the planned occlusal changes,[9] for Category 1 patients the use of such appliances is usually not considered to be necessary.[8] However, for patients with temporomandibular disorders, the use of a splint may still be advisable.[7]

For patients in this category, where a reconstructive approach is planned using *additive/minimal intervention*, the clinical techniques for applying adhesively retained restorations are akin to those described for the transfer of the information derived from the dental wax-up as per previous chapters.

When undertaking restorative rehabilitation for a case displaying generalised wear (regardless of the category), ideally half the increase in OVD should be incorporated into each arch, but the final decision often depends on the pattern of wear and the desired aesthetic outcome (e.g. the length of the upper incisors). Where the increase in OVD is shared equally between the dental arches, it may help to provide a more even distribution of the increase in crown to root ratio across the dentition and also render the increase in OVD less abrupt, thereby helping to improve the overall chances of successful adaptation.[8]

The decision to restore the anterior or posterior segment first is very much operator driven. Whilst some clinicians prefer to restore the anterior teeth first (offering the benefits of establishing an appropriate aesthetic outcome and anterior/canine guidance at the process of care delivery), others may chose to restore the posterior segments, to help control the occlusal form of the molar and premolar teeth (especially when trying to attain a group function occlusal scheme),[10] whilst also ensuring an adequate thickness and coverage of restorative material in the first instance.

Occasionally, it may also be decided to sequence the placement of restorations, such that either the anterior *or* posterior segments are restored in separate visits. This may prove to be less cumbersome for the operator and patient, as the treatment of one complete arch in a single phase can be highly challenging from a technical perspective. Phasing may also help with the distribution of treatment fees. Under such circumstances, where a stabilisation splint may have been initially provided, this can be sectioned (by the removal of aspects of the splint where the restorations have been fitted) to help ensure/improve the chances of the short-term survival of the newly placed restorations by providing some level of protection from excessive occlusal loads at the treatment segments). In more recent times, however, or where a splint may not have been prescribed, it has become commonplace to place centric stops in either glass ionomer cement or direct resin composite to help maintain the space created in the posterior segments.

Where *conventional restorations* are being planned (especially amongst cases where the existing clinical crown may be very short and composite resin restorations likely to respond in an unpredictable manner when exposed to higher occlusal loads), preliminary tooth preparations (of at least one arch) can be carried out in one single visit.[3] This will allow for the fabrication of the provisional restorations for all the teeth at the planned OVD. The choice of which arch to prepare first will depend on the occlusal plane discrepancy (usually the arch with the greatest discrepancy will be prepared first). Acrylic or silicone indices formed from the diagnostic wax-up may also prove beneficial in assisting the operator with the precise level of occlusal surface reduction required to accommodate the definitive restoration.[3,10]

The patient should be maintained in indirectly formed provisional restorations for a period of 6–8 weeks.[3,8] This time period will allow for an evaluation of the aesthetics and function as described in Chapters 6 and 13, respectively, but the length of this period will be mainly depend on the fabrication time of the indirect restorations. The provisional restorations may, however, require some adjustments. Once deemed acceptable, the provisional restorations may be used as an occlusal and aesthetic guide for the fabrication of the definitive restorations. The construction of a customised anterior guidance table can prove to be very beneficial (to copy the anterior occlusal scheme) as achieved with the use of the provisional restorations, where the anterior guidance has been shown to be mechanically acceptable. For further details see Chapter 6.

Where metallo-ceramic crowns are being prescribed, it may be worthwhile undertaking metal and/or biscuit try-in stages to minimise the risk of errors propagating during the undertaking of restorative care. The final occlusal scheme should aim to leave the patient with a mutually protected occlusion, as discussed above.

13.2.2 Category 2: Excessive wear without loss of OVD

In such cases, a discrepancy may be seen to exist between the inter-cuspal position (ICP) and the first point of tooth contact in centric relation (CRCP), thus space may be 'created' by the distalisation of the mandible towards CR. Whilst this may provide some level of inter-occlusal clearance (which may be utilised to accommodate the desired restorative materials), the amount of space yielded may not always be sufficient. Under such circumstances there may be a need to plan a concomitant increase in the OVD. For these cases, the traditional approach has been to prescribe patients with a full-coverage, hard acrylic occlusal splint, which will provide an increase in the OVD to the required range, whilst the mandible is concomitantly manipulated into its retrusive arc of closure.[8]

The occlusal prescription of the splint should aim to provide a removable mutually protective scheme, and the patient instructed to wear the splint continually for a period of 1 month (at all times other than when eating) to evaluate the tolerance of the increase in OVD.[11] Once the operator is satisfied that the patient can tolerate the planned occlusal changes, the process of preliminary tooth preparation may begin, in the manner as described for Category 1 patients. In certain cases, composite resin can be included anteriorly during the construction of the occlusal splint to allow for some aesthetic compensation during the evaluation stage.

Unpredictable compliance with splint therapy has prompted an alternative approach, as described by Vialati and Belser.[12] They described a protocol that involves the placement of indirect provisional resin composite onlay and/or palatal resin veneers at the same occlusal prescription as would be provided by a full coverage hard occlusal splint. This may also be done using direct resin composite, as illustrated by the clinical case in Figure 13.4.

In some cases, where an occasional tooth may not display significant wear, the decision may be taken to avoid restorative material placement and to allow for some occlusal adaptation to take place, with the longer-term goal of attaining the desired occlusal scheme.

13.2.3 Category 3: No Loss of OVD, with Insufficient Space for Restorative Materials'

Category 3 cases are considered to be the most taxing to restore as the required inter-occlusal space is not readily available. This is due to tooth repositioning as a consequence of alveolar compensatory growth. According to Rivera-Morales and Mohl,[8] in such cases every effort should be made to obtain space by *means other than an increase in the OVD*. Only if such methods fail to provide enough space would an increase in the OVD be advocated. This would be accomplished by the programmed modification of the OVD through the careful use of occlusal splints.

Other methods that can be used under such circumstances are described below:

13.2.3.1 Surgical Crown Lengthening, with Osseous Re-contouring

Although restoration margins may be placed subgingivally, ideally the restoration margin should be placed no more than 0.5 mm sub gingivally to prevent encroachment of the biological width. Where the latter is invaded, chronic periodontal inflammation with concomitant periodontal breakdown may follow, resulting in the re-establishment of the biological width in a more apical position. To avoid this, surgical crown lengthening is indicated.[13]

Surgical crown lengthening with osseous re-contouring can be used to increase the quantity of coronal tooth tissue, particularly in the case of teeth with short clinical crown heights, where further occlusal reduction may severely compromise retention and resistance from where conventional restorations are being planned. However, it is important for the patient to have a good standard of oral hygiene as well as to carry out a careful assessment of the periodontal tissues and the crown to root ratio, as the clinical technique involves the removal of 2–3 mm of alveolar bone, which may culminate in a mobile tooth in the case of a root with an unfavourable crown to root ratio.[10,14]

When planning cases, a diagnostic wax-up should be prepared where the effect of the surgical process is crudely copies onto a diagnostic cast and an intra-oral mock-up done accordingly to enable the patient to see the effect of crown lengthening surgery on the appearance of the definitive restorations. Careful consideration should also be given the position and symmetry of the gingival zeniths.[10,14]

Surgical crown lengthening may result in unsightly *black triangles* between the teeth and also lead to unfavourable crown to root ratios.[10] Gingival recession also often accompanies the healing process, which may result in the exposure of subgingival margins. Where possible, methods of tissue retraction and impression making should be carefully undertaken to help avoid damage to the supra-crestal attachment.[15]

It is also important to allow an adequate period of healing prior to the placement of definitive restorations (particularly in the anterior region) for the avoidance of poor post-restorative aesthetics and to allow the level of the gingival crest to stabilise.[15] A period of up to 6 months between the periodontal surgery and the placement of the definitive restorations has been advocated,[16] but it has also been suggested that an excessive delay in carrying out the latter processes may increase the risk of tissue rebound.[10]

Other drawbacks associated with crown lengthening include post-operative sensitivity, especially as the restorative margins will need to be placed up on newly exposed root dentine. Where the treated tooth has a marked coronal-cervical taper, this may also culminate in the need for a highly destructive preparation form, with the risk of pulpal complications.[17]

13.2.3.2   Elective Endodontics with Post-Placement

Elective endodontics may be considered to permit the application of a post and core system to further augment the available core material for the case of a grossly over-erupted tooth where there is a need to correct the occlusal plane discrepancy (where occlusal reduction would otherwise result in iatrogenic pulpal exposure) or for the preparation of a tooth to serve an overdenture.

Post-retained crown restorations are well known for their predisposition to failure by root fracture (especially where metallic post and core systems are used). This problem is likely to be compounded amongst patients who display severe bruxist tendencies.

Furthermore, the undertaking of elective endodontic therapy might also compromise the long-term prognosis of the affected tooth should root canal therapy prove to be unsuccessful. Under such circumstances, the full risks and benefits of elective endodontic treatment must be very carefully explained and evidence for the attainment of informed consent maintained. In the opinion of the authors, the use of post-retained crowns should be avoided where possible.

13.2.3.3   Orthodontic Tooth Movement

Orthodontic tooth movement[18] can be used to permit the intrusion of grossly over-erupted teeth or the extrusion of teeth with short clinical crowns (where there is a copious quantity of alveolar bone support), to provide intra-occlusal clearance by increasing the overjet and reducing the overbite, and may also help with the process of improving the alignment of the anterior dentition. However, the intrusion of selected teeth can prove to be an unreliable process with the concomitant risks of root resorption.[17]

13.3   Conclusions

Once restorative rehabilitation is indicated, meticulous treatment planning with due regard to the aesthetic and functional requirements is required along with the careful selection of materials. It is recommended that a stage in the planning is included which allows the patient to approve and visualise the intended final restorative prescription, particularly from an aesthetic point of view. Patient awareness of the adaptive mechanism and expectations is integral to treatment success.

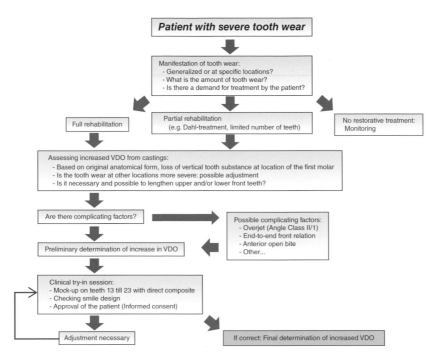

Figure 13.1 Flowchart to show the restorative management of patients with severe tooth wear.

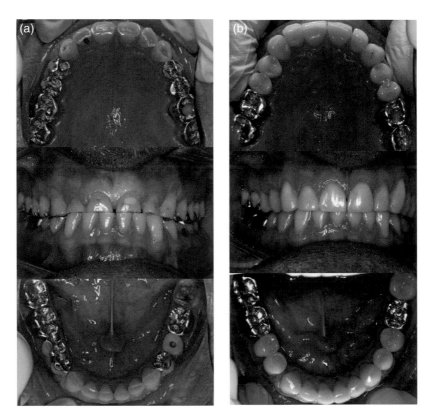

Figure 13.2 (a) Patient with generalised TW in the upper and lower arch where the posterior restorations are showing signs of failure and wear. (b) Patient as shown in (a) following full mouth rehabilitation and replacements of the failed posterior restorations at a long-term review appointment.

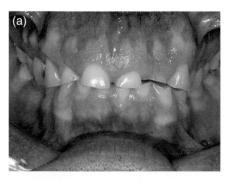
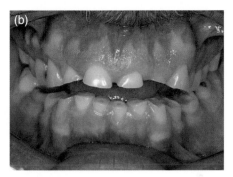

Figure 13.3 Patient with severe generalised TW.

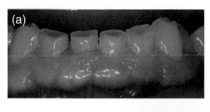
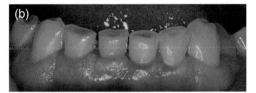
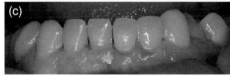

Figure 13.4 (a) Patient with TW on the lower anterior teeth. (b) Patient shown in (a) following periodontal crown lengthening. (c) Following periodontal crown lengthening for the anterior teeth for the patient shown in (a) and (b). Direct composite restorations have been placed. Image shows patient at a recall appointment.

References

1 Turner, K. and Missirilian, D. (1984). Restoration of the extremely worn dentition. *J. Prosthet. Dent.* 52: 467–474.

2 Loomans, B. and Opdam, N. (2018). A guide to managing tooth wear: the Radboud philosophy. *Br. Dent. J.* 224: 348–356.

3 Mehta, S.B., Banerji, S., Millar, B.J., and Saures-Fieto, J.M. (2012). Current concepts in tooth wear management. Part 3 Active restorative care 2: The management of generalised tooth wear. *Br. Dent. J.* 212 (3): 121–127.

4 Rosenstiel, S., Land, M., and Fujimoto, J. (2011). *Contemporary Fixed Prosthodotnics*, 3e. Mosby.

5 Hobkirk, J. (2009). Loss of the vertical dimension of occlusion and its management complications. *Int. J. Prosthodont.* 22: 520.

6 Morley, J. and Eubank, J. (2001). Macroesthetic elements of smile design. *J. Am. Dent. Assoc.* 132: 39–45.

7 Loomans, B., Opdam, N., Attin, T. et al. (2017). Severe tooth wear: European consensus statement on management guidelines. *J. Adhes. Dent.* 19: 111–119.

8 Rivera-Morales, W. and Mohl, N. (1993). Restoration of the vertical dimension of the occlusion in the severely worn dentition. *Dent. Clin. N. Am.* 36: 651–663.

9 Wassel, R., Steele, J., and Welsh, G. (1998). Considerations when planning occlusal rehabilitation: a review of the literature. *Int. Dent. J.* 48: 571–581.

10 Varma, S., Preisjel, A., and Bartlett, D. (2018). The management of tooth wear with crowns and indirect restorations. *Br. Dent. J.* 224: 343–347.

11 Gross, M. and Ormianer, Z. (1994). A preliminary study on the effects of occlusal vertical dimension increase on mandibular postural rest position. *Int. J. Prosthodont.* 7: 216–226.

12 Vialati, F. and Belser, C. (2008). Full mouth adhesive rehabilitation of a severely eroded dentition: the three step technique. Part 2. *Eur. J. Esthet. Dent.* 3: 128–138.

13 Briggs, P. and Bishop, K. (1997). Fixed prosthesis in the treatment of tooth wear. *Eur. J. Prosthodont. Restor. Dent.* 4: 175–180.

14 Patel, R. and Baker, P. (2015). Functional crown lengthening surgery in the aesthetic zone; periodontic and prosthodontic considerations. *Dent. Update* 42: 36–42.

15 Talbot, T., Briggs, P., and Gibson, M. (1993). Crown lengthening: a clinical review. *Dent. Update*: 301–306.

16 Wise, M. (1995, Chapter 20, Periodontal Surgery). *Failure in the Restored Dentition: Management and Treatment*, 317–334. Quintessence Books.

17 Yule, P. and Barclay, S. (2015). Worn down teeth by toothwear? Aetiology, diagnosis and management revisited. *Dent Update* 42: 525–532.

18 Evans, R. (1997). Orthodontics and the creation of localised inter-occlusal space in cases of anterior tooth wear. *Eur. J. Prosthodont. Rest. Dent.* 5: 169–173.

14

The Prognosis of the Restored Worn Dentition: Contingency Planning, the Importance of Maintenance, and Recall

14.1 Introduction

Patients with restored dentitions will need follow-up to determine the clinical performance of the restorations. If a worn dentition is restored, than the specific aetiology leading to the pathological condition may be a risk factor for survival of the treatment result. Ongoing erosive wear may disintegrate the marginal inter- face of restorations, leading to breakdown and restorations extending from the occlusal surface. Bruxing patients will impose high loading to a restoration, increasing the risk for fracture.[1,2] Therefore, despite preventive measures, such as the prescription of a nightguard, interventions are likely to occur in the years following the restorative treatment. Imperfections on restorations like dis- colorations, (chip-) fractures, wear, etc. are the main reasons for interventions.[3] Interventions may be simple procedures like polishing and refurbishment, but can be also be restorative interventions as repair or replacement of the restoration.

Complete replacement of failed restorations in dentistry is usually costly and time-consuming. Defective dental restorations can be replaced, but nowadays repair can be considered as the gold standard treatment option.[4–7] In dentistry, repair can be described as replacing the failed or broken part of a restoration with a new one whilst leaving the intact part of the restoration in place. When a restoration fails as a result of imperfections like discoloration, microleakage, ditching at the margins, delamination, or simple fracture, there may be a need for repair or replacement. Partial replacement (repair) is often preferable. This can be achieved by adding a new layer of composite onto an existing one using appropriate bonding techniques. Repair includes a limited risk for complications and reduced loss of sound tooth substance compared to complete replacement. Given that every replacement would lead to a larger preparation size, repairs may slow down the so-called restorative cycle.[8]

For adhesion of composites to substrates other than tooth substance, a number of surface conditioning methods have been developed over the years using physical, physico-chemical, or chemical adhesion principles. Surface roughening is achieved using airborne particle abrasion, lasers, and etching agents such as acidulated phosphate fluoride, hydrofluoric acid, and phosphoric acid, whilst chemical conditioning methods involve the use of silane coupling agents and/or intermediate adhesive resins.[7,9]

Practical Procedures in the Management of Tooth Wear, First Edition. Subir Banerji, Shamir Mehta, Niek Opdam and Bas Loomans.
© 2020 John Wiley & Sons Ltd. Published 2020 by John Wiley & Sons Ltd.
Companion website: www.wiley.com/go/banerji/toothwear

Using repair techniques, the service life of defective restorations can be prolonged.[10,11] Advances in adhesive technologies have introduced several surface-conditioning concepts to bond resin composites onto different indirect and direct restorative materials (Figure 14.1). The aim of this chapter is to summarise reasons for failure and survival of restorations placed in patients with severe tooth wear (TW). Moreover, different concepts of repair techniques are presented, including the available surface conditioning methods as practical guidelines for intraoral repair procedures.

14.2 Survival of Direct and Indirect Restorations

14.2.1 Direct Restorations

In restorative dentistry, the most commonly used materials are amalgam and composite resin. In terms of clinical survival for posterior restorations, both materials show good long-term results and the mean annual failure rates vary between 1 and 3% after 10 years of service (Figure 14.2).[12–14] For amalgam and composite restorations the main reasons for failure are (secondary) caries and fracture of the restoration and tooth (Figure 14.3). However, clinical survival of dental restorations is a complex issue and depends on:

- the properties of the restorative materials[15]
- specific patient-related risk factors, such as:
  - oral hygiene
  - caries susceptibility[14]
  - bruxism[16]
  - the dentist.[17]

The presence of these patient-related risk factors may increase the probability of failure up to four times.[14] It is remarkable that in many clinical trials high-risk patients are often excluded, resulting in an inclusion bias in these studies. Consequently, the outcome of clinical trials may not always be representative of the general population. Failures of posterior composite restorations are often related to secondary caries and fracture of the restoration.

14.2.2 Indirect Restorations

From a systematic review, with a mean follow-up time of 7.3 years, an annual failure rate was reported for metal-ceramic single crowns of 0.88, resulting in estimated survival after 5 years of 95.7%.[18] All-ceramic crowns had an annual failure rate ranging between 0.69 and 1.96, resulting in an estimated survival rate between 90.7 and 96.6%. Various all-ceramic crowns showed different survival rates. When compared with metal-ceramic crowns early types of feldspathic/silica-based ceramics and zirconia crowns presented statistically significant lower 5-year survival rates of 90.6 and 91.2%, respectively. In contrast, lithium-disilicate reinforced glass ceramics (estimated 5-year survival of 96.6%), glass-infiltrated alumina (estimated 5-year survival of 94.6%), and densely sintered alumina (estimated 5-year survival of 96.0%) were comparable to metal-ceramic crowns. For metal-ceramic crowns, ceramic chipping was the most frequent technical complication, with a cumulative 5-year event rate of 2.6% (95% confidence interval [CI], 1.3–5.2%) (Figure 14.4). For all-ceramic crowns a tendency to more chipping of the veneering ceramic was observed for alumina- and zirconia-based single crowns than for all other ceramic crowns. Fractures of the framework were rarely found with metal-ceramic crowns, whereas this was significantly more often found for all-ceramic crowns. A problem specifically found more for zirconia crowns was loss of retention.[18]

Failure of ceramic restorations (crowns, veneers, onlays, and inlays) seems also to be related to individual risk factors. A 2.3 times greater risk of failure was found in patients with existing parafunctional habits.[19] Another study found that parafunctional habits resulted in statistically significant increased chipping of the veneering ceramic.[20]

The results presented on the clinical longevity of direct and indirect restorations are based on clinical studies including patients without severe TW and therefore these results cannot be directly transferred to patients treated with severe TW. As a matter of fact, in many clinical studies on indirect restorations, patients with signs of bruxism were excluded.[21] Therefore, it may be expected that results on longevity of direct and indirect restorations as published in the literature are not valid for the specific high-risk group of TW patients.

14.3   Repair and Replacement

The majority of restoration fractures occur supragingivally, indicating that in most cases repair of the fractured teeth is not difficult and can be achieved with a direct composite restoration.[22] When these restorations are repaired, there is minimal intervention to tooth structure compared with a total replacement. Moreover, repair is more cost-effective than replacement of the whole restoration. Repair can be considered beneficial when it increases the longevity of dental restorations. As for repair of direct restorations, in a systematic review the Cochrane Collaboration evaluated the effects of repair versus replacement in the management of defective amalgam and composite restorations.[23,24] Unfortunately, no published randomised controlled clinical trial relevant to this review question could be identified. Because there is no clear consensus in the literature regarding when a failed restoration should be repaired or replaced, the best scientific evidence available is currently derived from several retrospective and prospective clinical trials and *in vitro* studies. In fact, repair is mainly indicated for localised shortcomings of restorations that are no longer clinically acceptable. Repair is a minimally invasive approach that implies the addition of a restorative material, not only glaze or adhesive, with or without a preparation in the restoration and/ or dental hard tissues. Replacement of the restoration is indicated if multiple or severe problems and intervention needs are present and a repair option is not reasonable or feasible. Repair procedures are not always without risk because sometimes extension in the preparation is necessary, which may yield iatrogenic (pulp) damage and make the treatment complex and costly. Furthermore, little information is available for general dental practitioners on the decision regarding when to repair or replace a failed restoration.

For successful repair, a durable bond has to be established between the old restoration and the new repair material.[7] Adequate surface conditioning of the substrate, selection of the adhesive resin, and restorative material are therefore prerequisites. In order to provide sufficient attachment to old and aged restorations, surface conditioning may be realised by macro-mechanical or micro-mechanical retention and/or chemical adhesion. Whereas macro-mechanical retention can be achieved by creating retention holes, undercuts, or simply roughening the surface with a coarse diamond bur, micro-mechanical retention is created by etching (e.g. phosphoric acid or hydrofluoric acid) or air abrasion with alumina or alumina particles coated with silica particles. In addition, a chemical bond may be established between resin and inorganic filler particles by application of special primers such as silane coupling agents.

14.4 Repair Techniques

14.4.1 Acid Etching

Etching of substrates is typically achieved by phosphoric acid or hydrofluoric acid. Phosphoric acid is effective on enamel and dentin but has no direct effect on surface characteristics of composites, ceramics, and metals. However, etching has a beneficial effect on retention rates after repair due to a cleansing and degreasing effect on these surfaces.[25] Unlike phosphoric acid, hydrofluoric acid dissolves glass particles present in ceramics, and in most of the composites leaves the resin matrix unaffected. Because fewer inorganic filler particles are present in microfine composites, the effect of etching with hydrofluoric acid in this type of composite is particularly limited. Therefore, it is important to realise that the effect of hydrofluoric acid is largely dependent on the composition of the filler particles in the material. Composite resins containing zirconium clusters or quartz fillers, for instance, will react less upon hydrofluoric acid etching than on composite resins consisting of barium-glass fillers.[25] The broad diversity of new materials requires the evaluation of their compatibility with respect to repairing ability. Unfortunately, often the history and type of failed composite could not be identified clinically unless it had been recorded in the patient's file.

When using hydrofluoric acid intraorally, direct contact with enamel and dentin as well as skin or mucosa should be avoided. On dentin and enamel a precipitate of calcium fluoride (CaF_2) is formed. This precipitate of CaF_2 can then prevent the infiltration of adhesive resin in the opened dentin tubuli, resulting in poor adhesion of composite to the contaminated enamel or dentin.[26,27] Contamination of the skin or mucosa with hydrofluoric acid is painless but may result in tissue necrosis in the deeper layers of the tissue.[28] To date, no side effects or negative reactions of hydrofluoric acid have been described in the dental literature.[29]

There is much uncertainty on the optimal concentration of hydrofluoric acid and the most effective duration of etching. A number of *in vitro* studies have dealt with this matter with a wide variety of materials and methods, making results difficult to compare directly.[9] Nevertheless, the general conclusion is that prolonged etching time does not necessarily result in better adhesion. Depending on the ceramic type and the composition of the glass matrix, prolonged etching time may remove glass particles from the surface, yielding to a less than optimum roughness and a decreased wettability of the subsequent silane coupling agent.

14.4.2 Air Abrasion/Sandblasting

Airborne-particle abrasion is typically applied using chairside air abrasion devices for intraoral repairs operating under a pressure between 2 and 3 bars. The substrate material to be conditioned, metal, ceramic, composite, or amalgam, is abraded for approximately 10 seconds from a distance of approximately 10 mm to achieve a clean and rough surface. The abrasion particles consist of aluminium oxide particles with a size of 30–50 µm or aluminium oxide particles coated with a silicon-dioxide layer, where the latter is referred as silicoating or tribochemical surface conditioning.[30] Alumina or silica particles coat the surface, which then make covalent bonds through the siloxane layer with the silane coupling agent. Given that one disadvantage of air abrasion is the aerosol with abrasive particles, a good suction device is mandatory to prevent aspiration of these particles.

14.4.3 Silane Coupling Agents

Following air abrasion, chemical adhesion can be established using special primers or monomers that react with the surface of a material.[31] The most common primer is a silane coupling agent that is also used in the fabrication of composites to adhere the inorganic filler particles chemically to the resin matrix. In dentistry, usually 3-methacryloxypropyltrimethoxysilane (MPS) is used, which is a bifunctional molecule. MPS silanes consist of, on one side, a methacrylate group that can react with the intermediate adhesive resin and composites, and, on the other side, a reactive silanol group that can form siloxane bonds with the alumina and/or silica present on the air-abraded or etched substrate surfaces. Silane coupling agents are presently available in two types, either hydrolysed or non-hydrolysed. The hydrolysed silanes are directly ready for use and should be applied as a separate step in the bonding procedure before the adhesive resin is applied. The non-hydrolysed silane has to be activated first with an acid, usually an acidic monomer (e.g. 10-methacryloyloxydecyl dihydrogen phosphate, 10-MDP), which is present in the primer or adhesive resin. Depending on the adhesive system, the silane coupling agent has to be mixed with the primer or adhesive resin. *In vitro* studies showed significant positive effects of the use of silane coupling agents in composite or ceramic repairs compared with those situations where no silane was used.[32]

14.4.4 Intermediate Adhesive Resins

Application of adhesive resin on the silanised surface increases the wettability of the composite to be used as the repair material. The effect of different substrate materials for composite–composite repair varies strongly, and it is generally advisable, but not compulsory, to combine identical composite materials.[33] Unfortunately, in most clinical situations the general practitioner does not know the composition of the failed restoration. Adhesion to glassy matrix ceramics is well established by hydrofluoric acid etching, silanisation, and adhesive resin application. Identical results for the repair of indirect composite restorations were found in which the use of airborne particle abrasion followed by a silane coupling agent adhesive resin resulted in the best surface conditioning.[34]

14.4.5 Clinical Protocols

Because clean surfaces are essential for adequate adhesion, the substrate surfaces need to be cleaned with fluoride-free prophylaxis paste prior to conditioning procedures. Thereafter, the appropriate physico-chemical surface conditioning method should be applied to the corresponding substrate type. Different intraoral repair protocols are presented to help the general practitioner to chose the optimal repair procedure.[7]

Ceramic fractures in metal-ceramic fixed dental prostheses:

1) Clean both the ceramic and metal surface using fluoride-free paste or pumice.
2) Remove glaze of the veneering ceramic surface at the margins to be repaired using a fine-grit diamond bur under water cooling and create a bevel.
3a) Air abrade the metal surface using only a chairside air abrasion device, wash and rinse under copious water, and dry thoroughly. Etch the ceramic margins where the repair composite will be adhered with 5% or 9.6% hydrofluoric acid (HF) for 20–90 seconds, depending on the manufacturer's instructions. Rinse for at least 60 seconds and dry.

or

3b) If intraoral use of HF is not desired, air abrade the ceramic surface and metal surface using a chairside air abrasion device, wash and rinse under copious water, and dry.
4) Apply silane coupling agent on both the metal and the ceramic surface (one layer) and dry gently.
5) If necessary, mask the metal surface with opaque resin and photopolymerise.

6) Apply adhesive resin on the veneering ceramic, air dry, and photopolymerise.
7) Apply resin composite incrementally, photopolymerise, finish, and polish the repair composite.

Fractures of composite resin restorations:

1) Clean the composite surfaces using fluoride-free paste or pumice.
2) Roughen the composite restorations at the margins to be repaired using a fine-grit diamond bur under water cooling and create a bevel.
3a) Etch the composite margins where the repair composite will be adhered with 5% or 9.6% HF for 20–90 seconds, depending on the manufacturer's instructions. Rinse for at least 60 seconds and dry.

or

3b) Air abrade the composite surface using a chairside air abrasion device, wash and rinse under copious water, and dry.
4) Apply silane coupling agent on composite surface (one layer) and dry gently.
5) Apply adhesive resin on the composite surface, air dry, and photopolymerise.
6) Apply resin composite incrementally, photopolymerize, finish, and polish the repair composite.

Fractures in zirconia fixed dental prostheses:

1) Clean both the veneer and zirconia surface using fluoride-free paste or pumice.
2) Remove glaze of the veneering ceramic surface at the margins to be repaired using a fine-grit diamond bur under water cooling and create a bevel.
3a) Air abrade the zirconia surface using only a chairside air abrasion device for approximately 20 seconds, wash and rinse under copious water, and dry thoroughly. Then etch the ceramic margins where the repair composite will be adhered with 5% or 9.6% HF for 20–90 seconds, depending on the manufacturer's instructions. Rinse for at least 60 seconds and dry.

or

3b) Air abrade both the zirconia and ceramic surface using a chairside air-abrasion device, wash and rinse under copious water, and dry.
4) Apply silane coupling agent on both the zirconia and the ceramic surface (one layer) and dry gently.
5) Apply adhesive resin on the zirconia and ceramic, air dry, and photopolymerise.
6) Apply resin composite incrementally, photopolymerise, finish, and polish the repair composite.

14.5   Conclusions

Repair of restorations that fail for technical reasons or due to fatigue could certainly prolong the survival of functioning restorations. The least minimally invasive and most cost-effective method should be chosen. Some minor defects around margins, such as minor discoloration or ditching, may not result in impaired function, and thus such failures could be only monitored instead of repaired or replaced.

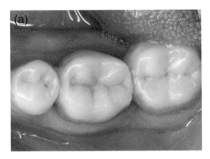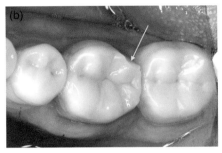

Figure 14.1 (a) Lava Ultimate indirect placed on the lower first and second molar teeth. (b) Failure (arrowed) of the restoration on the lower first molar shown in (a) at 1 year.

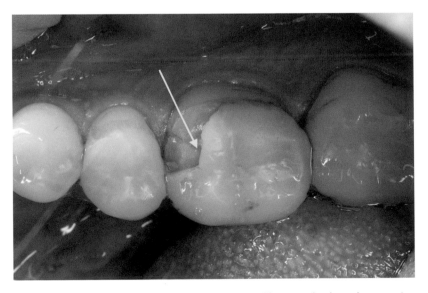

Figure 14.2 Patient with generalised TW in the upper and lower arch where the posterior restorations are showing signs of failure and wear (arrowed).

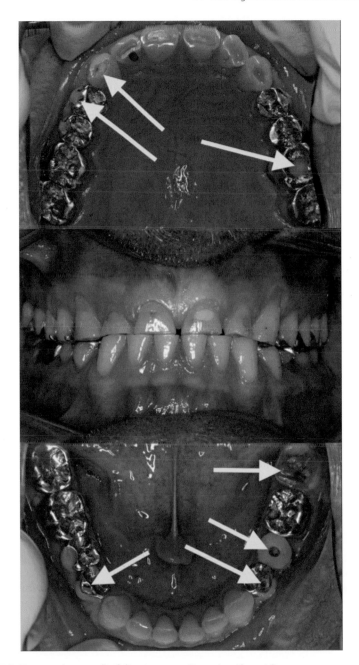

Figure 14.3 Fracture (arrowed) of direct composite restoration at 3 years.

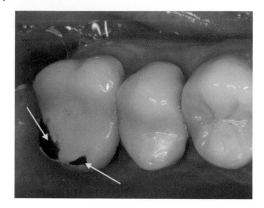
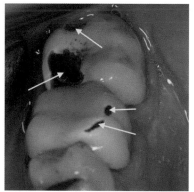
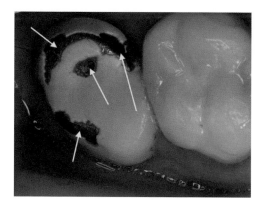

Figure 14.4 Ceramic fractures (arrowed) and failure of indirect metal ceramic crowns.

References

1 Van de Sande, F.H., Opdam, N.J., Rodolpho, P.A. et al. (2013). Patient risk factors' influence on survival of posterior composites. *J. Dent. Res.* 92: 78S–83S.
2 Van de Sande, F.H., Collares, K., Correa, M.B. et al. (2016). Restoration survival: revisiting Patients' risk factors through a systematic literature review. *Oper. Dent.* 41: S7–S26.
3 Loomans, B.A.C., Kreulen, C.M., Huijs-Visser, H.E.C.E. et al. (2018). Clinical performance of full rehabilitations with direct composite in severe tooth wear patients: 3.5 years results. *J. Dent.* 70: 97–103.
4 Mjör, I.A. (1993). Repair versus replacement of failed restorations. *Int. Dent. J.* 43 (5): 466–472.
5 Mjör, I.A. (2005). Clinical diagnosis of recurrent caries. *J. Am. Dent. Assoc.* 136 (10): 1426–1433.
6 Hickel, R., Roulet, J.F., Bayne, S. et al. (2008). Recommendations for conducting controlled clinical studies of dental restorative materials. *Clin. Oral Investig.* 11: 5–33.

7 Loomans, B. and Özcan, M. (2016). Intraoral repair of direct and indirect restorations: procedures and guidelines. *Oper. Dent.* 41: S68–S78.

8 Elderton, R.J. (1990). Clinical studies concerning re-restoration of teeth. *Adv. Dent. Res.* 4 (1): 4–9.

9 Loomans, B.A., Cardoso, M.V., Roeters, F.J. et al. (2011). Is there one optimal repair technique for all composites? *Dent. Mater.* 27 (7): 701–709.

10 Casagrande, L., Laske, M., Bronkhorst, E.M. et al. (2017). Repair may increase survival of direct posterior restorations – a practice based study. *J. Dent.* 64: 30–36.

11 Opdam, N.J., Bronkhorst, E.M., Loomans, B.A., and Huysmans, M.C. (2012). Longevity of repaired restorations: a practice based study. *J. Dent.* 40 (10): 829–835.

12 Heintze, S.D. and Rousson, V. (2012). Clinical effectiveness of direct class II restorations – a meta-analysis. *J. Adhes. Dent.* 14 (5): 407–431.

13 Opdam, N.J.M., Bronkhorst, E.M., Loomans, B.A.C., and Huysmans, M.C.D.N.J.M. (2010). 12-year survival of composite vs amalgam restorations. *J. Dent. Res.* 89 (10): 1063–1067.

14 Opdam, N.J., van de Sande, F.H., Bronkhorst, E. et al. (2014). Longevity of posterior composite restorations: a systematic review and meta-analysis. *J. Dent. Res.* 93 (10): 958–985.

15 Demarco, F.F., Corrêa, M.B., Cenci, M.S. et al. (2012). Longevity of posterior composite restorations: not only a matter of materials. *Dent. Mater.* 28 (1): 87–101.

16 van de Sande, F.H., Opdam, N.J., Rodolpho, P.A. et al. (2013). Patient risk factors' influence on survival of posterior composites. *J. Dent. Res.* 92 (7): S78–S83.

17 Laske, M., Opdam, N., Bronkhorst, E. et al. (2016). Ten-year survival of Class II restorations placed by general practitioners. *JDR Clini. Transl. Res.* 1 (3): 292–299.

18 Pjetursson, B.E., Sailer, I., Zwahlen, M., and Hammerle, C.H.F. (2007). A systematic review of the survival and complication rates of all-ceramic and metal-ceramic reconstructions after an observation period of at least 3 years. Part 1: Single crowns. *Clinl. Oral. Impl. Res.* 18 (3): 73–85.

19 Beier, U.S., Kapferer, I., and Dumfahrt, H. (2012). Clinical long-term evaluation and failure characteristics of 1,335 all-ceramic restorations. *Int. J. Prosthodont.* 25 (1): 70–78.

20 Koenig, V., Vanheusden, A.J., Le Goff, S.O., and Mainjot, A.K. (2013). Clinical risk factors related to failures with zirconia-based restorations: an up to 9-year retrospective study. *J. Dent.* 41 (12): 1164–1174.

21 Opdam, N.J.M., Collares, K., Hickel, R. et al. (2018 Jan). Clinical studies in restorative dentistry: new directions and new demands. *Dent. Mater.* 34 (1): 1–12.

22 Fernández, E.M., Martin, J.A., Angel, P.A. et al. (2012). Survival rate of sealed, refurbished and repaired defective restorations: 4-year follow-up. *Braz. Dent. J.* 22 (2): 134–139.

23 Sharif, M.O., Merry, A., Catleugh, M. et al. (2014). Replacement versus repair of defective restorations in adults: amalgam. *Cochrane Database Syst. Rev.* (2): CD005970.

24 Sharif, M.O., Catleugh, M., Merry, A. et al. (2014). Replacement versus repair of defective restorations in adults: resin composite. *Cochrane Database Syst. Rev.* (2): CD005971.

25 Loomans, B.A.C., Cardoso, M.V., Opdam, N.J.M. et al. (2011). Surface roughness of etched composite resin in light of composite repair. *J. Dent.* 39 (7): 499–505.

26 Pioch, T., Jakob, H., García-Godoy, F. et al. (2003). Surface characteristics of dentin experimentally exposed to hydrofluoric acid. *Eur. J. Oral Sci.* 111 (4): 359–364.

27 Loomans, B.A.C., Mine, A., Roeters, F.J.M. et al. (2010). Hydrofluoric acid on dentin should be avoided. *Dent. Mater.* 26 (7): 643–649.

28 Asvesti, C., Guadagni, F., Anastasiadis, G. et al. (1997). Hydrofluoric acid burns. *Cutis* 59 (6): 306–308.

29 Özcan, M., Allahbeickaraghi, A., and Dündar, M. (2012). Possible hazardous effects of hydrofluoric acid and recommendations for treatment approach: a review. *Clin. Oral Investig.* 16 (1): 15–23.

30 Edelhoff, D., Marx, R., Spiekermann, H., and Yildirim, M. (2001). Clinical use of an intraoral silicoating technique. *J. Esthet. Restor. Dent.* 13 (6): 350–356.

31 Swift, E.J. Jr., Cloe, B.C., and Boyer, D.B. (1994). Effect of a silane coupling agent on composite repair strengths. *Am. J. Dent.* 7 (4): 200–202.

32 Filho, A.M., Vieira, L.C., Araújo, E., and Monteiro Júnior, S. (2004). Effect of different ceramic surface treatments on resin microtensile bond strength. *J. Prosthodont.* 13 (1): 28–35.

33 Baur, V. and Ilie, N. (2013). Repair of dental resin-based composites. *J. Adh. Dent.* 17 (2): 601–608.

34 Souza, E.M., Francischone, C.E., Powers, J.M. et al. (2008). Effect of different surface treatments on the repair bond strength of indirect composites. *Am. J. Dent.* 21 (2): 93–96.

Index

Practical Procedures in the Management of Tooth Wear, First Edition. Subir Banerji, Shamir Mehta,
Niek Opdam and Bas Loomans.
© 2020 John Wiley & Sons Ltd. Published 2020 by John Wiley & Sons Ltd.
Companion website: www.wiley.com/go/banerji/toothwear